AF605152

Dr Daniel Golshevsky

Dr Daniel Golshevsky (Dr Golly) is a Melbourne-based paediatrician and father of three.

As a general paediatrician, Dr Golly cares for babies, children and teenagers of all ages, managing physical, mental and behavioural development as well as illnesses and emergencies.

While Dr Golly's primary focus outside of clinic has been newborn and toddler sleep, as his profile has grown, so too have calls for him to help families with general illness and common childhood conditions.

Dr Golly's philosophy remains centred around empowering parents. In a world of infinite and unchecked resources, he is passionate about creating content for parents that is easy to understand, from a trusted source.

Background and education:

- Bachelor of Medicine, University of Melbourne, Australia
- Fellow of the Royal Australasian College of Physicians
- Former Chief Resident Medical Officer of The Royal Children's Hospital, Melbourne, Australia

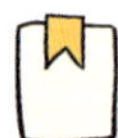

Proud:

- Red Nose Australia Ambassador
- Clinical Perinatal Mental Health Champion of the Gidget Foundation
- Professional Member of the Australian Breastfeeding Association
- Peer-reviewed author on pediatric sleep and obesity
- International clinical practice guidelines reviewer
- General pediatric trainee lecturer

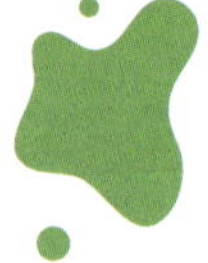

Find him on socials @drgolly

Learn more: drgolly.com

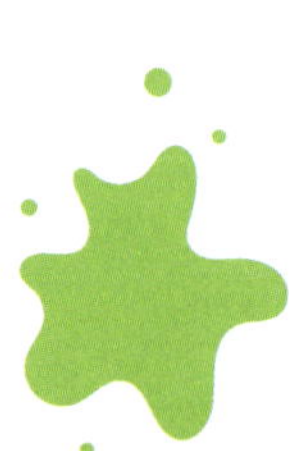

Dr Golly's GUIDE TO FAMILY ILLNESS

Sneezes, Wheezes and Common Diseases

Hardie Grant acknowledges the Traditional Owners of the Country on which we work, the Wurundjeri People of the Kulin Nation and the Gadigal People of the Eora Nation, and recognises their continuing connection to the land, waters and culture. We pay our respects to their Elders past and present.

Hardie Grant Children's Publishing
Wurundjeri Country
Level 11, 36 Wellington Street
Collingwood Victoria 3066
Melbourne | Sydney | San Francisco

hardiegrant.com/childrens

ISBN: 9781761215339
First published 2025

Image credits: *HFMD pg. 125* reproduced with permission from ©DermNet 2025, Shutterstock, Inc/Jang's Studio, TANAPAT LEK.JIW, Pao_saman2008 *Chickenpox pg. 128* Shutterstock, Inc/RHJPhtotos, Inc *pg. 129* Shutterstock, Inc/almo Creative, Nenad Nedomacki *Slapped cheek pg. 133* Shutterstock, Inc/Yevhen Prozhyrko, then reproduced with permission from ©DermNet 2025 *Cold sores pg. 136* Shutterstock, Inc/C.PIPAT *pg. 137* Shutterstock, Inc/OMfotovideocontent, Victoria 1 *Measles pg. 140* Shutterstock, Inc/Natalya_Maisheva *pg. 141* Shutterstock, Inc/fotohay *Meningococcal disease pg. 145-6* both reproduced with permission from ©DermNet 2025 *HSP pg. 149* all reproduced with permission from ©DermNet 2025 *School sores (impetigo) pg. 154* Shutterstock, Inc/Zay Nyi Nyi, FotoHelin, reproduced with permission from ©DermNet 2025, Dr Golly Sleep Program PTY LTD *Molluscum pg. 158* Joaquin Corbalan P, reproduced with permission from ©DermNet 2025 *Scabies pg. 161* Shutterstock, Inc/Zay Nyi Nyi *pg. 162* Shutterstock, Inc/ Sapan Unhale, Paosun Rt *Eczema pg. 165* Shutterstock, Inc/Aisylu Ahmadieva,marishkaSm, Alyona Shu, Ruslan Ivantsov *Oral thrush pg. 194* Shutterstock, Inc/Victoria 1 *Ringworm (tinea) pg. 204* Shutterstock, Inc/sruilk *pg. 205* Shutterstock, Inc/Zay Nyi Nyi, Raylog, Zay Nyi Nyi, muroPhotographer *Warts pg. 208* reproduced with permission from ©DermNet 2025 *Acne pg. 231* Shutterstock, Inc/KHON SUPAN, Nau Nau, DUANGJAN J, me2724, Bencemor, gnepphoto **Rash table**: as above, and *Acne (newborn) pg. 238*, reproduced with permission from ©DermNet 2025 *Cutis marmorata pg. 239*, reproduced with permission from ©DermNet 2025 *Hives pg. 240*, Shutterstock, Inc/FotoDuets, nidchita, TANAPAT LEK.JIW, Arlee.P *Milia pg. 241*, reproduced with permission from ©DermNet 2025 *Miliaria pg. 241*, reproduced with permission from ©DermNet 2025 *Nappy rash pg. 242*, reproduced with permission from ©DermNet 2025 *Roseola infantum pg. 242*, Shutterstock, Inc/wk1003mike, Jes2u.photo, justkgoomm, NeoStudio1 *Scabies pg. 242*, reproduced with permission from ©DermNet 2025

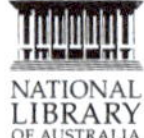

A catalogue record for this book is available from the National Library of Australia

Publisher Marisa Pintado
Design Hannah Schubert
Editorial Penelope White, Emma Schwarz with Claire Davis
Production Amanda Shaw
Illustrator Cora Muccitelli

Printed in China by Leo Paper Group

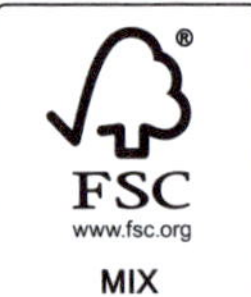

The paper this book is printed on is certified against the Forest Stewardship Council® Standards and other sources. FSC® promotes environmentally responsible, socially beneficial and economically viable management of the world's forests.

2 4 5 3 1

Dr Golly's GUIDE TO FAMILY ILLNESS

Sneezes, Wheezes and Common Diseases

Dr Daniel Golshevsky

PAEDIATRICIAN

Hardie Grant

BOOKS

This book is dedicated to the unsung heroes of healthcare – nurses.

Your tireless work on the frontlines, keeping children safe and healthy, is an inspiration. As a paediatrician, I witness your unwavering compassion and skill every day. To quote Maya Angelou: 'They may forget your name, but they will never forget how you made them feel.' Thank you for making our children feel safe, loved and cared for.

– Dr Golly

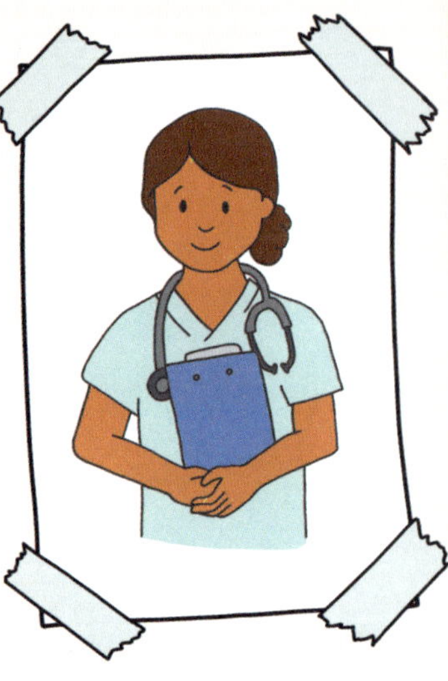

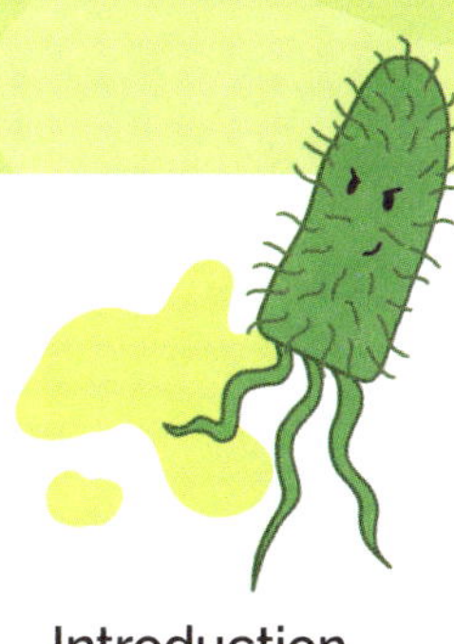

Contents

Childcare BINGO!

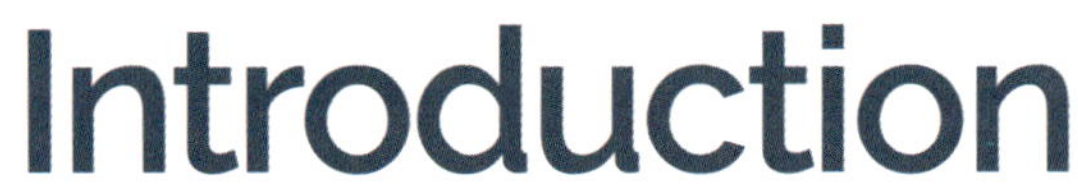

Introduction

I'm Dr Golly, paediatrician and father of three.

For more than a decade, parents have told me of their frustration with deciphering online information regarding their baby and children's health. They worry in the middle of the night when their child is unwell, second-guess their parental instincts and lose sleep fretting about common childhood infections and conditions. This book isn't medical advice. It is designed to be your quick-reference guide for the most common symptoms and signs you're likely to encounter along the wonderful rollercoaster we call parenthood. **When our children are uncomfortable, we are uncomfortable.** While we strive to alleviate our children's symptoms and get them well as soon as possible, I hope that this book empowers and comforts parents too. We need it just as much!

As your children move around the community, it's inevitable they'll pick up a few bugs, or lurgies, along the way. It can be really tough to know when to see a doctor and when you can just let them rest up. This resource is your go-to guide: it will help you navigate through many of the most common illnesses, prepare basic management plans and, most importantly, identify severe illness, when you may need more support. I've also included some of the most googled health topics that parents want to learn about.

This book isn't a diagnostic tool and it's not medical advice. My hope is that it prepares you for many of the common illnesses that you're likely to encounter, and alerts you to the less common, but critical, illnesses that you need to be able to recognise quickly – using a trusted resource.

An important note on our medical systems:

Medical staff are here to serve our communities – whether they're Nurse-On-Call, maternal child health nurses, general practitioners (GPs), paediatricians and other specialists, paramedics or emergency departments. While this book is designed to empower parents and reduce unnecessary anxiety, there are times when the medical system is needed. In these cases, don't ever hesitate. The medical system works in tandem with you – parents, carers and guardians – so if you have a child who needs care, your role is to seek this help when needed.

Trust your parental instincts

Parents have an extraordinary sixth sense when it comes to knowing something is not right with their child. I urge you to listen to – and trust – these instincts. You'll notice a constant theme throughout this book: *if something doesn't feel right, have your child reviewed by a healthcare professional.*

Dr Golly

PAEDIATRICIAN

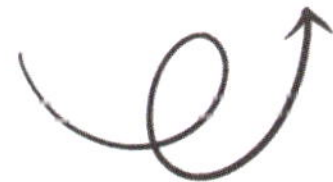

"

Parents can often feel like their young children are spinning on a merry-go-round of almost-constant illness. This is normal, and I'm here to help.

"

General sickness 101

What to do when your child is sick, and how to tell if it's an emergency

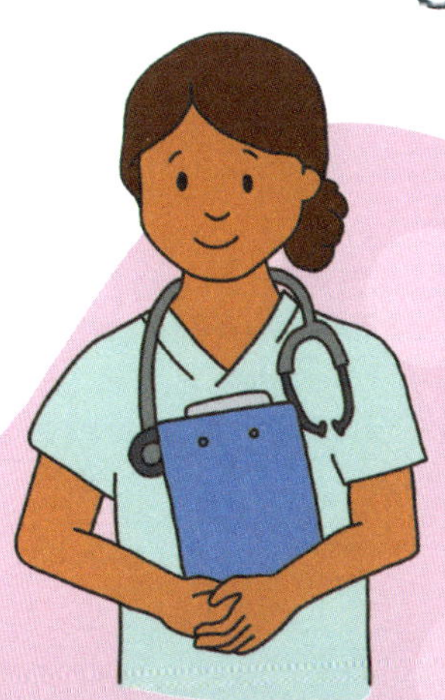

A CHILDHOOD SICKNESS IS INEVITABLE!

We can minimise it, but not avoid it completely

We can do our very best to stay healthy – by practising great hand hygiene, staying hydrated, prioritising sleep, eating well-balanced diets, minimising viral spread and staying up to date with immunisations – but we cannot avoid family illness completely. Especially when our children are young.

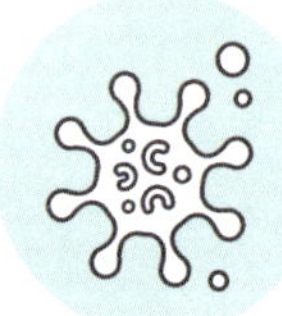

In fact, many parents feel that their child is always sick, especially if the child goes to childcare or kindergarten. That's understandable! It is normal for healthy children in a childcare setting to experience a viral infection once a month. That's a dozen infections a year ... and they can linger! While the symptoms of a viral cold in children are usually mild and last between seven and ten days, it's common for a cough to hang around for up to three weeks (for a happy, recovered child).

Do the maths: one week of a cold plus three weeks with a lingering cough equals a month, and the next virus is just around the corner! It can often feel like you're on a merry-go-round, with the impression of **almost-constant illness**.

The good news is that the sickness merry-go-round doesn't last forever. As your child develops, and they don't play on the ground as much – bringing fewer objects to their mouth – they won't get sick as often.

In the meantime, it's essential that you are empowered and prepared with basic management plans and a clear sense of when to seek expert advice. In this section, we will cover what to do when you realise your child is unwell, and the most common symptoms you'll see at home.

Despite the sickness merry-go-round, I am a big supporter of utilising childcare! While a group care setting exposes children to more bugs – and a higher frequency of infections – it also offers a lot of advantages.

As well as allowing parents to work or have time to themselves, group care offers our kids socialisation, growth and development – not to mention opportunities to learn the fundamentals from highly skilled childcare educators (think toilet and sleep training). It's wonderful on so many levels.

MYTHS and FACTS

Myth: My child will have to be exposed to germs at some point. If they don't go to childcare they'll be sicker when they start school.

Fact: While a child's immune system does improve with age as they approach adulthood, children who attend childcare do not have a more powerful immune system than those who remain at home until they start school; this is a myth. We'll talk about this more in the section on **colds** (page 76) but by the time kids are five or six years old, both their hygiene and the way they play has changed, so the frequency of infection drops dramatically.

What to keep at home

It's a good idea to keep a supply of items at home to help you in triaging and managing illness in your family. This isn't a family first-aid kit – that would need many more items – but it does cover all the essential items we regularly reference throughout this book.

Keep on hand:

- saline (spray, drops or ampoules)
- nasal aspirator
- oral rehydration solution
- a quality digital thermometer
- fever-reducing medication
  - paracetamol
  - ibuprofen
- printouts of illness trackers.

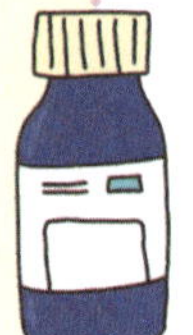

Keep up to date:

- immunisation schedule
- ambulance insurance, if required.

Ambulance call-outs without insurance can be expensive. You can purchase ambulance insurance for your family, and most private health insurers include it in their policy cover. If there's an emergency, you'd never want to think twice about providing critical care for your child because of the cost. Healthcare, pension and disability cardholders are often eligible for free ambulances without insurance – check your state guidelines.

Who you can call for help

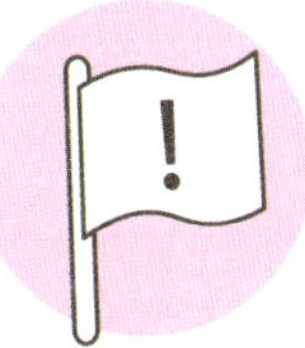

When assessing your child's illness, my advice – as always – is to trust your parental instincts. When in doubt, always seek medical help.

If you need support to know what to do next, you can use the following resources (remember they may differ depending on where you live):

1. Call a Nurse-On-Call telephone service.
2. Call a maternal child health nurse.
3. See your local doctor or GP.
4. See your paediatrician.
5. Call an after-hours GP service (home-visiting or telehealth).
6. Go to an emergency department (ED), in person or online.
7. Call an ambulance.

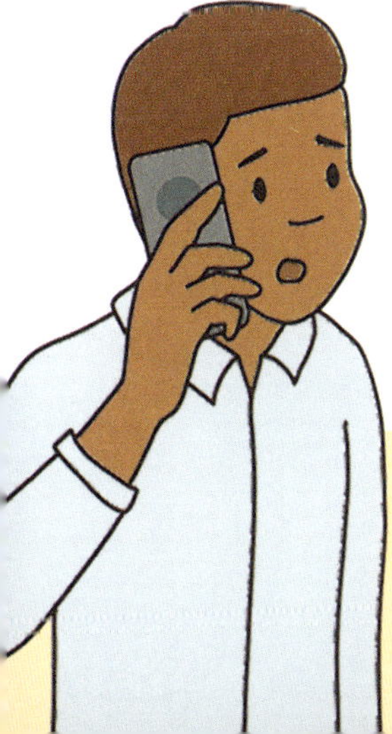

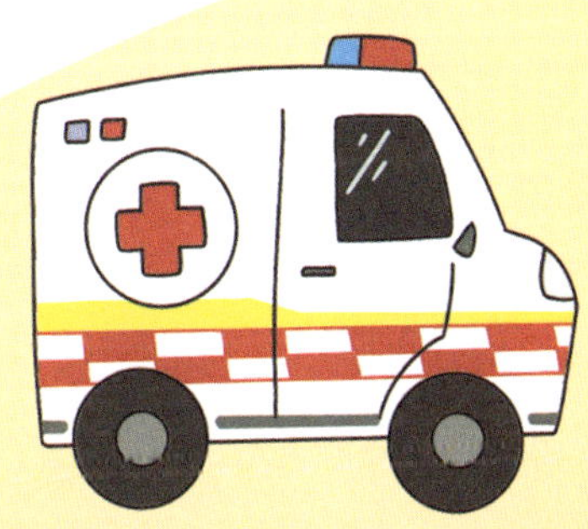

Warning signs of severe illness

Most parents know what to do in an emergency, but the more complicated question is: how do you know when it IS an emergency? A child's condition can change quickly and a mildly sick child can deteriorate with little warning. Children also may not clearly explain how they are feeling, which can make it harder to identify a medical problem and treat it quickly.

One framework to help guide you through this quandary is the **3B and 3P quick-assessment tool**. You can use this as a quick-reference, first-step checklist when you realise your child is unwell.

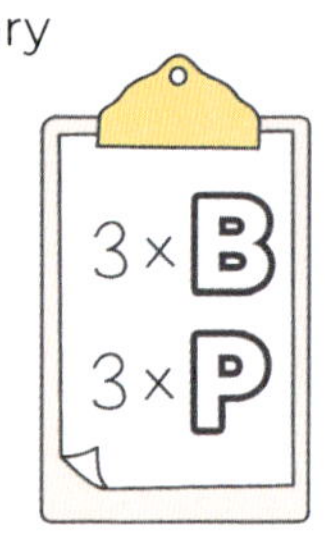

No matter what the illness or issue, the **3Bs** and **3Ps** will help you understand when your child needs urgent medical care, and when it's something that can wait until the morning. If your child shows any of these warning signs, seek medical attention.

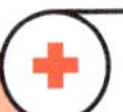

SEEK URGENT MEDICAL HELP

Non-blanching rashes

It doesn't fit neatly into the **3B** and **3P** tool, but a **non-blanching rash** – in other words, a rash that doesn't turn white when you press on it – is very serious and needs immediate medical attention. See more on page 36.

Remember: If in doubt, always take your child to a medical professional.

The 3 Bs

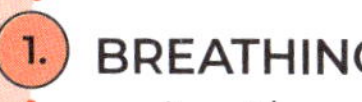

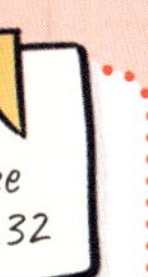

1. BREATHING:

- Are they working hard to breathe?
- Are they breathing faster or noisier?

2. BEHAVIOUR:

- Has their behaviour changed in any way, or are they acting strangely?
- Are they really difficult to wake or unusually drowsy?

3. BREAST AND BOTTLES:

- What is happening with their fluid intake? This includes their usual intake, such as breastmilk and formula for younger babies, and water for older children, as well as oral rehydration solution and icy poles.
- If they are drinking less than 50 per cent of their usual intake, or refusing to drink any fluids, this is a red flag.

The 3 Ps

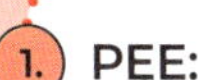

1. PEE:

- Are there fewer wet nappies than usual?
- Is the urine concentrated – very yellow and/or foul-smelling?
- For older children, are they taking fewer trips to the toilet?

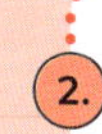

2. POO AND VOMIT:

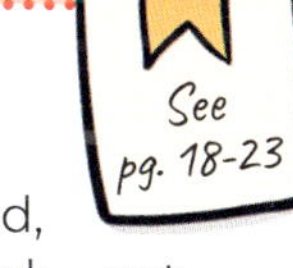

- If you see red, white or black – get it checked.

3. PAIN:

- Are they having increasing or persistent pain?
- Are they having eye pain or headache when exposed to light (photophobia)?
- Is there pain associated with fever and/or breathing difficulties?

If you answered yes to any of these questions, seek medical attention immediately.

Collecting samples for your doctor

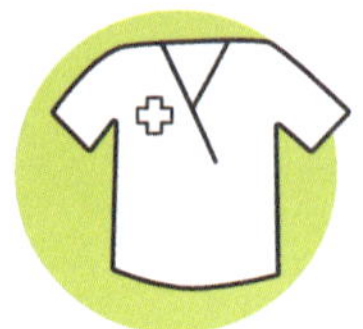

A doctor may request various scans and samples so they can investigate further. The most common of these are requests for urine and poo samples. For older children, collecting both urine and poo samples can be straightforward, as poo samples are for babies using nappies. But collecting urine samples for babies and younger children can be a challenge for many parents.

Firstly, ask your doctor if the sample needs to be 'sterile' or not. A doctor might also provide a sterile device – a urine bag – that can safely be attached to the skin to collect urine. If your attempts fail, a doctor or nurse can insert a catheter, or they may insert a small needle directly into the bladder (this is called suprapubic aspiration).

Sterile urine collection

Clean the child before collecting the sample then, using gloves, catch the urine halfway through the stream, making sure there is no contamination.

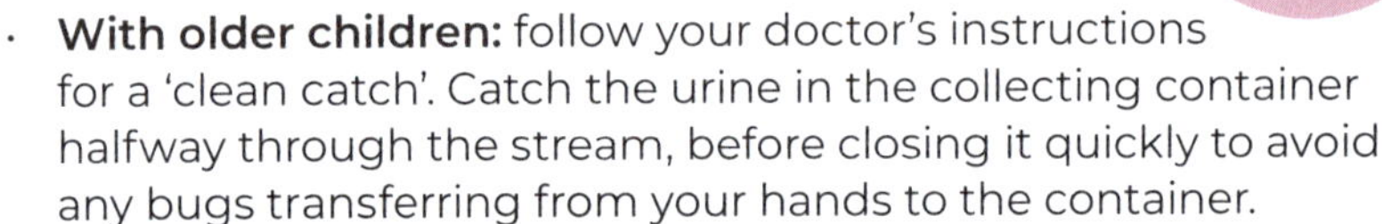

- **With older children:** follow your doctor's instructions for a 'clean catch'. Catch the urine in the collecting container halfway through the stream, before closing it quickly to avoid any bugs transferring from your hands to the container.
- **With younger children:** lie them on their back and remove their nappy. When a urine stream begins, try to catch some of the urine in the middle of the stream.

Non-sterile urine collection

Hydrate your child. If a urine bag has been provided, place it on the child's skin. If not, insert some cotton-wool balls into the nappy. Once soaked, these cotton-wool balls can be squeezed directly into a sample container.

TIP

Collecting urine can be a hysterical, frustrating task that might take hours – and multiple streams of urine! You can stimulate urination by wiping a wet cloth on your child's lower abdomen.

Fever

First-aid kit items:

- thermometer
- fever-reducing medication

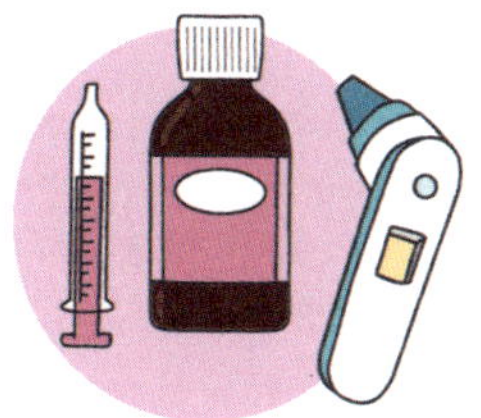

Fever is one of the most common reasons parents bring their children to see me, and understandably so. It can be scary when your little one's temperature rises, but it's important to understand that fever is not an illness in itself – it's a sign that the body is fighting an infection.

What is the normal temperature range for children?

The normal temperature for children is between 36°C and 37.5°C, although this can vary according to the time their temperature is taken, the method of checking and the device used.

What is fever?

Fever – often called a 'febrile episode' by doctors – is defined as a core body temperature that's above the normal range, typically above 38°C. However, it's important to note that normal body temperature can vary slightly from child to child, at different ages, and even throughout the day.

To accurately measure your child's temperature you'll need a reliable thermometer. There are various types available, including digital and traditional oral, rectal, ear and forehead thermometers.

When an infection starts, signalling proteins travel through the body to alert the immune system. These proteins also alter the body's natural thermostat, turning it down. This means that the body feels cold, even though it's at normal temperature. So the body works to increase the body's temperature in an attempt to correct the thermostat. That's why we feel cold, despite being hot to touch.

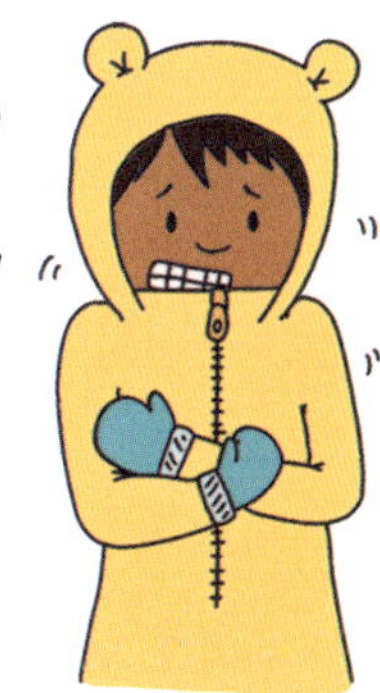

What causes a fever?

A fever is most commonly caused by an infection, such as a cold or flu, an ear infection or a urinary tract infection (UTI). It can also be a reaction to certain vaccinations or medications, or from inflammation (swelling). In rare cases, fever may be a sign of a more serious underlying condition.

While very high temperatures are definitely concerning, doctors pay more attention to the 'trend' of medium–high temperatures as opposed to the absolute number.

What happens when your child is between 37.5°C and 38°C?

Some childcare centres have a fever policy that anything over 37.5°C is considered a fever, prompting your child to be sent home. Some parents give fever-reducing medication as soon as the thermometer is over 37.5°C.

If your child is showing no signs of illness other than simply a number on the thermometer, my first piece of advice would be to remove a layer of their clothing and offer them a drink of water in a cool, quiet space. If their temperature goes down, it was probably just a sign that they were hot. If their temperature is trending up it's probably a sign that they are fighting something. There is a general push in healthcare to move away from measuring the exact number as there is so much variance in thermometers. The trend, environment and other symptoms are what to look for.

That said, if a baby under three months has a temperature over 37.5°C, always have them reviewed by a doctor immediately.

Recognising fever in children

Aside from an elevated temperature, other common signs of fever in children include:

- warm or flushed skin
- sweating
- chills or shivering
- irritability or fussiness
- decreased appetite
- lethargy or sleepiness.

When fever is a concern

While fever is usually a normal response to illness, there are certain situations when you should seek medical attention promptly.

Infants under three months old:

- Any fever in this age group is abnormal. Low temperature is also of concern – as is temperature instability (moving from high to low rapidly). Any concerns in this age group require immediate medical review.

High fever:

- A fever above 38.5°C (101.3°F) may need to be evaluated by a doctor, especially if accompanied by other symptoms.

Persistent fever:

- A fever lasting more than three to five days, regardless of the temperature, should be checked by a doctor.

Concerning symptoms:

- If your child has a fever along with difficulty breathing, a stiff neck, severe headache, a rash, confusion or any other worrying sign, seek medical attention.

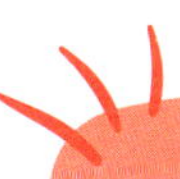

For any of these situations, seek medical attention immediately.

Managing fever at home

In most cases, mild fevers can be managed at home with supportive care.

Hydration:

- Encourage your child to drink plenty of fluids, such as water, breastmilk or formula, rehydration solution or even diluted juice. This helps prevent dehydration, which can make them feel worse. Breastfed babies can be offered more frequent feeds, older babies (older than six months) can have their regular fluid intake supplemented with water and oral rehydration solutions.

Comfort measures:

- Dress your child in light clothing and keep the room at a comfortable temperature. You can use a damp face washer on their forehead to help them feel comfortable.

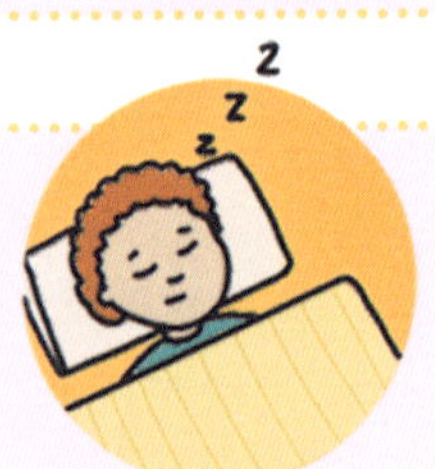

Fever-reducing medications:

- Over-the-counter medications like paracetamol or ibuprofen can help reduce fever and relieve discomfort. Always follow the recommended dosage for your child's age and weight, and consult your doctor or pharmacist if you have any questions.

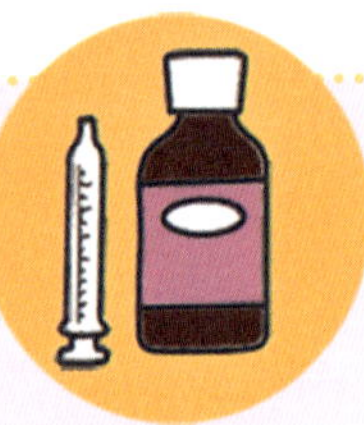

Remember: There is no need to 'treat the fever' if your child is happy. Having a mild fever is not dangerous and if your child is perfectly comfortable and hydrated, there is no need for fever-reducing medication. Remember to always treat the child, not the number.

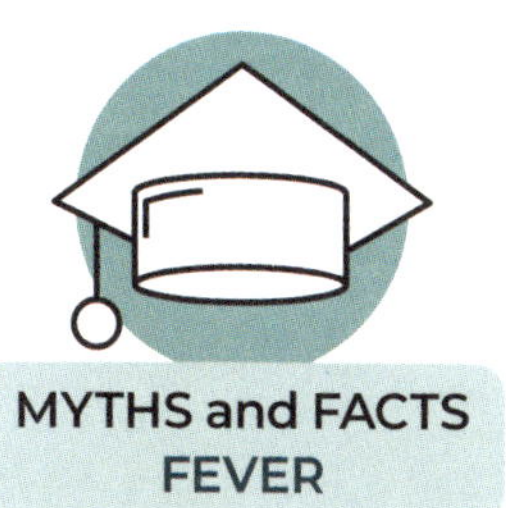

MYTHS and FACTS FEVER

Myth: A high fever will cause brain damage.

Fact: Fevers that occur with common childhood illnesses rarely cause brain damage.

Myth: All fevers are dangerous and need to be treated immediately.

Fact: Most fevers are a normal response to infection and help the body fight off illness.

Myth: It's important to 'break a fever'.

Fact: In some cultures, patients are intentionally overheated to treat a fever. This does not work and is potentially dangerous.

Myth: You need to cool down a feverish child using wet towels, cold baths and no blankets.

Fact: Children can become hypothermic (too cold) when over-cooled to reduce a fever. Dabbing their face with a wet washer may help, but trying to cool the entire body is not advised and will probably make your child more uncomfortable.

Remember: Fever is a common childhood symptom, and most fevers resolve on their own with supportive care.

Many of the illnesses throughout this book will feature fever as a common symptom. No matter what's causing the fever, how you manage it will often be the same.

If you're ever concerned about your child's fever or overall health, don't hesitate to reach out to your local doctor. We're here to help you navigate through any health concerns and ensure your child receives the best possible care.

Dehydration

This is one of the most common presentations to the emergency department in a paediatric hospital when a child is unwell. It is often a doctor's primary concern.

Mild dehydration may present as:

- dry lips, mouth or tongue
- a reduction in wet nappies or trips to the toilet
- nausea
- headaches
- a concentrated urine colour (it will look darker yellow and may have a strong smell)
- thirst (if your child is thirsty, they are already dehydrated).

Severe dehydration may present as:

- a sunken fontanelle, for a baby (the soft spot on a baby's skull)
- sunken eyes, absent tears
- floppiness, listlessness
- lethargy
- extreme thirst
- pale, cold hands
- lace pattern on the skin
- fast breathing.

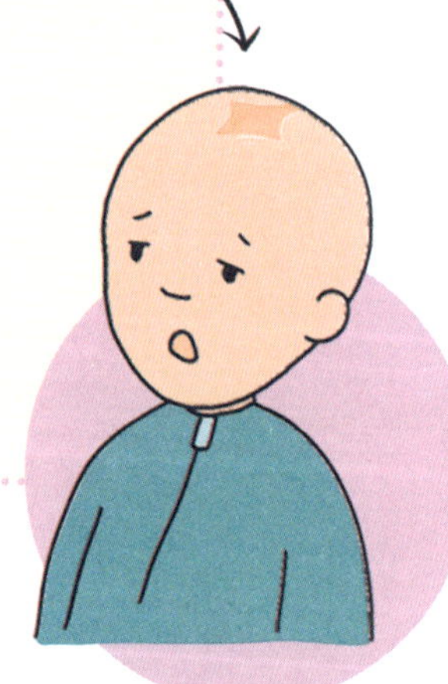

If your child is dehydrated, don't worry if they don't eat properly for a few days. They will eat when they are hungry. Fluids are crucial for survival. Your child needs fluid for bodily functions; food can wait.

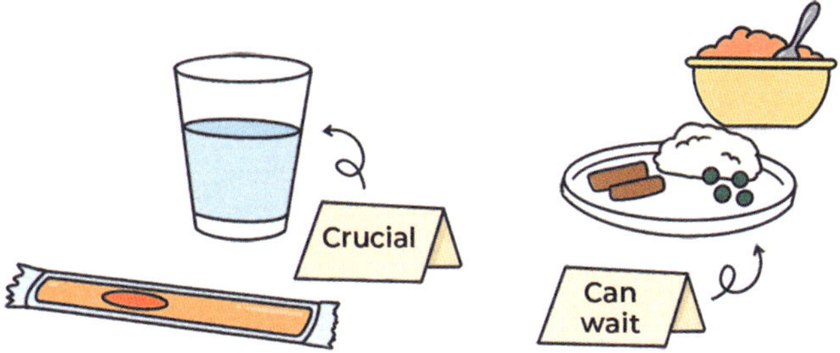

Dehydration prevention and treatment tips:

- If your child is younger than six months, they should always have a medical review when dehydrated.
- For babies over six months, rehydration is important:
  - Continue breastfeeding, and offer the breast more often.
  - Oral rehydration solutions and water can be given for the first twelve hours.
  - Syringes are a great way to deliver oral rehydration solutions – you can do 5–10 ml at a time.
  - If formula feeding, replace feeds with oral rehydration solution or water for the first twelve hours, then revert to formula – give smaller volumes more frequently.
  - If you are not comfortable managing this at home, seek medical attention.
- For older children, over twelve months:
  - Give oral rehydration solution in a syringe.
  - Offer rehydration ice blocks.
  - If your child won't take a rehydration solution you can use diluted apple juice – 50/50 with water for a short time only (any fluid is better than no fluid).
  - Try small volumes, more often.
  - Give your child sips of water every fifteen minutes when they are awake.
  - If you can get your child to drink a cup of water every hour for four hours, this is helpful.

Vomit

Vomiting is a common symptom of many childhood illnesses and, while it can be alarming for parents, it's not always a major cause for concern. Let's explore the common reasons children vomit, how to manage it at home, and when it might be time to seek medical attention.

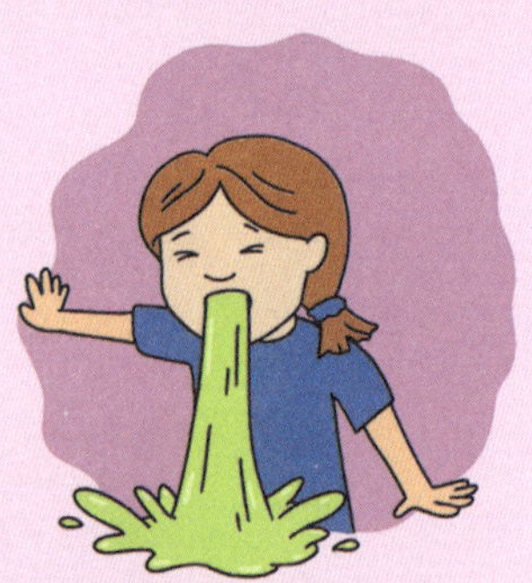

What causes vomiting in children?
The list of potential culprits is long, but here are some of the most common reasons:

- **Viral gastroenteritis ('gastro' or stomach flu):** This is a common viral infection of the stomach and intestines that causes vomiting, diarrhoea, abdominal cramps and sometimes fever (we'll talk more about this on page 71).
- **Food poisoning:** Eating contaminated food can trigger vomiting, diarrhoea and stomach cramps.
- **Motion sickness:** Travelling by car, boat or plane can make some kids feel nauseous.
- **Overeating or eating too quickly:** Sometimes, a tummy that's too full just needs to empty itself. Being overly active after a meal can also cause vomiting. Children should never swim immediately after eating.
- **Head injury:** Vomiting can sometimes be a symptom of a concussion or other head injury.
- **Other infections or inflammation:** Ear infections, urinary tract infections (UTIs) and even appendicitis can cause vomiting.
- **Medication side effects:** Some medications can trigger nausea and vomiting.
- **Intestinal blockage:** In rare cases, vomiting can be a sign of a blockage in the intestines, which requires urgent medical attention.

Vomiting in babies is a bit different, because babies spill milk – this is often described as vomit but it might not be. All babies bring up milk, but not every spit-up is a true vomit.

Broadly speaking, there are four ways milk comes up:

1. **Posset:** This is a small, effortless ejection of milk known as a posset (and is relevant for smaller babies). These cause no distress, no weight loss, no issues at all and are not concerning if the baby is thriving.

2. **Vomit:** This is an ejection of the stomach contents, involving retching/gagging and the movement of other muscles, like the shoulders lifting up. This will empty the stomach and, yes, this milk needs to be replaced. Large vomits occurring infrequently are not problematic, but recurrent vomiting needs to be investigated.

3. **Projectile vomit:** This is caused by an obstructed stomach, most often caused by pyloric stenosis (an uncommon condition in infants that blocks food from entering the small intestine). This is unmissable – the vomit will hit the ceiling or the wall behind you, and worsens quickly. Projectile vomiting is a medical emergency.

4. **True reflux:** Gastro-oesophageal reflux disease is an uncommon condition, in which stomach acid flows back up into the oesophagus. This leads to feed refusal, poor growth, bloody vomits, irritability and a chronic cough. This needs to be reviewed by a doctor.

Recognising the signs: is it just a posset?
For infants, occasional spit-ups (possets) after feeding is normal. However, vomiting is different – it's usually more forceful and involves larger amounts of stomach contents, as well as muscle involvement (sometimes referred to as heaving).

See pg. 9

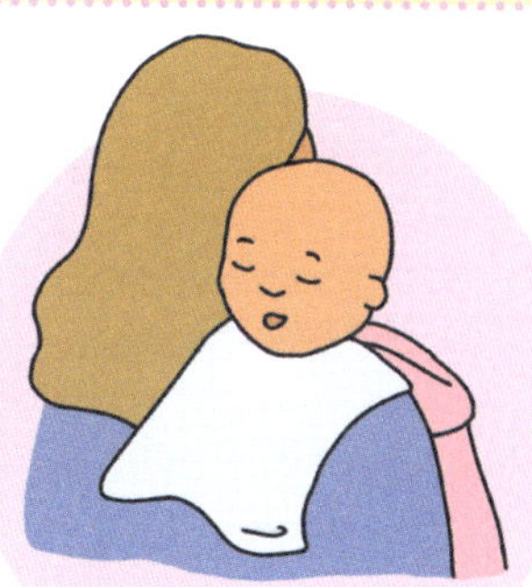

Signs of vomiting in older children can include:

- retching or gagging before or during vomiting
- abdominal pain or discomfort
- nausea
- loss of appetite.

Managing vomiting at home in children over six months: tips for relief

Most episodes of vomiting in children are caused by viruses and resolve on their own within a few days. Here's how you can help your child feel better at home:

1. **Rest:** Encourage your child to rest and avoid strenuous activity.

2. **Hydration:** Offer small, frequent sips of clear fluids like water, oral rehydration solutions or broth. Avoid sugary drinks and dairy.

3. **Bland foods:** Once the vomiting has stopped, start with small amounts of bland and developmentally appropriate foods, like toast, crackers or rice. Gradually reintroduce their regular diet as they tolerate it.

4. **Avoid strong odours:** Strong smells can trigger nausea, so keep the environment calm and odour-free.

5. **Medication:** Over-the-counter medications for nausea and vomiting may be helpful, but always consult your doctor before giving any medication to your child.

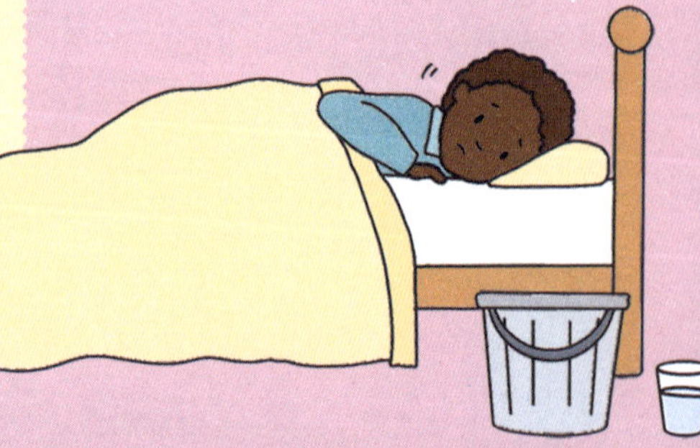

SEEK MEDICAL HELP

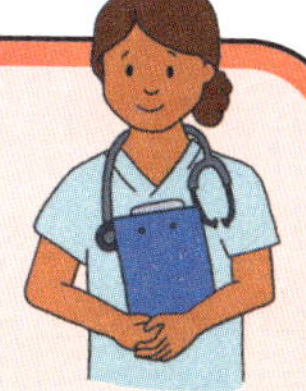

While most vomiting episodes are self-limiting, here are some signs that you should seek medical attention:

1. severe dehydration (signs of dehydration include dry mouth, sunken eyes, decreased urine output and lethargy)
2. blood in the vomit or stool
3. severe abdominal pain
4. high fever that doesn't respond to medication
5. projectile vomiting
6. bright green vomit colour (bile)
7. signs and history of a head injury
8. vomiting that lasts more than twenty-four hours (in children) or twelve hours (in infants)
9. vomiting that occurs with a rash, stiff neck or other concerning symptoms
10. the child is under six months of age.

A word of reassurance

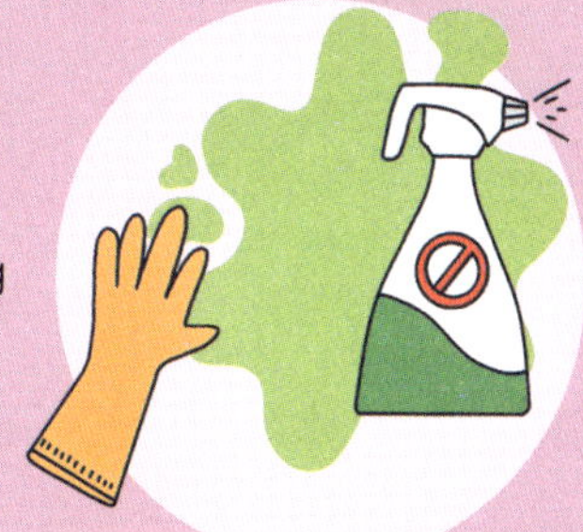

Vomiting can be a messy and unpleasant experience, but it's usually a sign that the body is trying to rid itself of something that's upsetting the stomach. By providing supportive care, ensuring adequate hydration and monitoring your child's symptoms, you can help them recover comfortably. While caring for your child, remember to protect yourself as much as possible: ensure strict hand hygiene, use gloves, wear a mask and disinfect contaminated surfaces, toys or utensils. If you have any concerns, don't hesitate to reach out to your local doctor.

Poo

The number of poo pictures that I receive as a paediatrician would amaze you! Whether it's for a baby or an older child, poo gives good insights into several things that might be going on with your child. In this section we'll look at what poo consistency, texture, frequency and colour can tell us about a child's overall health.

Consistency:

- Stringy, shiny mucus can be a sign of gut intolerance in babies. See your doctor if your baby has mucus in their poo.
- Explosive, frothy poo may be a sign of lactose overload in breastfed babies who are fed too often.
- For older children, runny poo can be a sign of a gastro virus or other illness.

Frequency:

- For breastfed babies, frequency can vary from seven times a day to one poo every seven days.
- Frequency is more of a question for older children.
- We'll discuss constipation specifically over the page.

Seek medical attention if the child has a gastro-type bug and:

- they're having more than eight to ten runny poos in a day, or
- they haven't improved after forty-eight hours.

Poo colours of concern:

The main colours to remember are black, red or white. If you see any of these colours, take your child to the doctor.

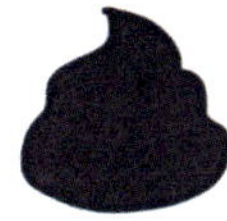

Black

Meconium passed in a baby's first few days is black (very dark green), but your baby's poo should not stay black in colour once meconium passes. Black poo can be a sign that your baby has ingested some blood or might be bleeding from higher up in the gastrointestinal tract; it is not normal. Sometimes, if the child is breastfeeding, the blood is from cracked and bleeding nipples.

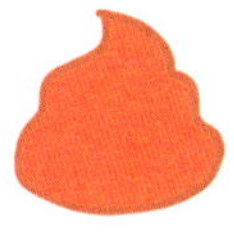

Red

This is not normal and could be a sign of bleeding. It can also be a sign that your baby has an intolerance.

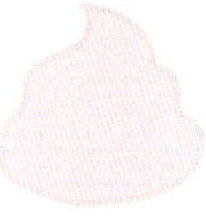

White

This is not normal. It could be a sign that the liver and gallbladder system aren't working correctly, making the poo white in appearance, with a chalky texture.

Other poo colours to be aware of:

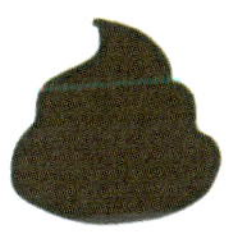

Dark green or greenish black

Meconium passed in the first few days. This is your baby's first poo and is sticky and tar-like. It is a combination of amniotic fluid, bile and fatty acids that your baby ingested while still in the womb.

Mustard yellow

Normal breastfed baby poo; pasty or seedy. Breastfed babies can also have looser brown or green poo.

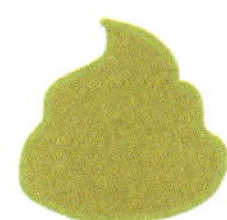

Light green

Normal formula-fed baby poo; it has simply passed through your baby's gut faster.

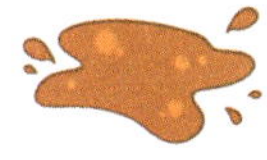

Pasty light brown

Normal poo for babies on formula, with a peanut-butter consistency.

Thick brown

Normal poo once solid foods are introduced, that resembles more of an adult poo, with a stronger smell than when just on milk feeds.

Constipation

I often encounter concerns about constipation in children. While it's a common issue, it can be unbelievably distressing for both kids and parents.

What is constipation, really?
Constipation isn't just about infrequent bowel movements. It's a broader issue that involves poo consistency, the difficulty of passing a poo, and associated symptoms like abdominal discomfort or bleeding.

A good rule of thumb is that if your child has fewer than three bowel movements a week, and those movements are hard, dry or difficult to pass, they are probably constipated.

Why do kids get constipated? Let's delve into the common culprits behind constipation in children.

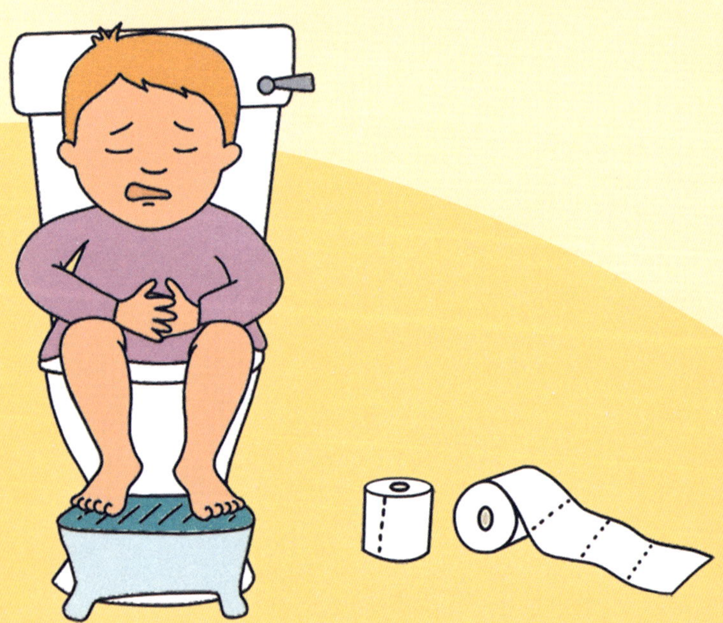

1. **Diet:** Fibre is like a scrub brush for the digestive tract, helping to bulk up stool and keep things moving. If your child's diet lacks fibre-rich foods like fruits, vegetables and whole grains, they're more likely to experience constipation. Additionally, inadequate fluid intake can dehydrate stool, making it harder to pass.

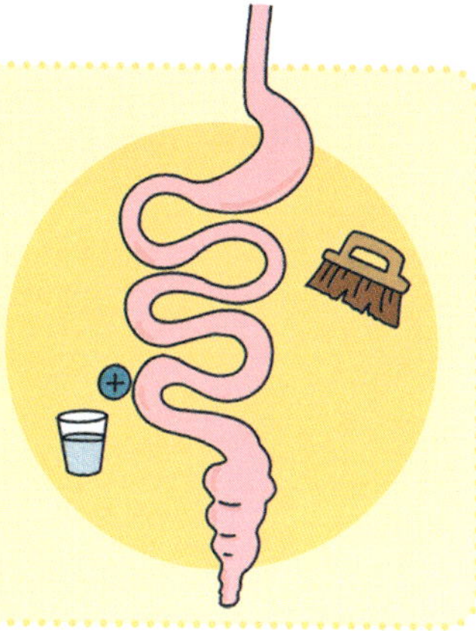

2. **Withholding:** Sometimes, children ignore the urge to pass a bowel action. They might be too engrossed in play, afraid of using the toilet, or experiencing discomfort due to an earlier bowel movement. This can create a vicious cycle, as holding it in further hardens the stool.

3. **Toilet-training troubles:** Anxiety or resistance during toilet-training can lead to withholding, and then constipation. If your child feels pressured or stressed about using the toilet, they might hold back their poo.

4. **Medical conditions:** While less common, certain underlying medical conditions can contribute to constipation. These include anatomical issues, like Hirschsprung's disease, endocrine or metabolic conditions, connective tissue disease, and neurological disorders. Medications may also contribute, as is commonly the case with iron supplementation. If your child isn't responding to simple treatment methods, or you suspect a medical cause, consult your doctor.

Recognising the signs: beyond infrequent stools

Besides the obvious infrequent bowel movements, here are some subtle signs that might indicate constipation:

- **Stomach pain:** This is often described as cramping or a dull ache in the lower abdomen.
- **Feeling full or bloated:** Your child might complain of feeling full, even after eating a small amount.
- **Decreased appetite:** They might not be interested in eating as much as usual.
- **Hard, pebble-like stools:** Small poo that resembles rabbit droppings is constipation.
- **Straining and discomfort during bowel movements:** This can be distressing for children and lead to fear of using the toilet.
- **Soiling:** This involves leaking small amounts of stool into underwear, usually due to impacted stool in the rectum.
- **Blood:** Painful passage and bright-red blood upon wiping are often indicative of a fissure – a small tear – in the anal sphincter. This occurs commonly in constipation and is extremely painful.

Helping your child: practical tips and tricks

Fortunately, there are many ways to help your child overcome constipation:

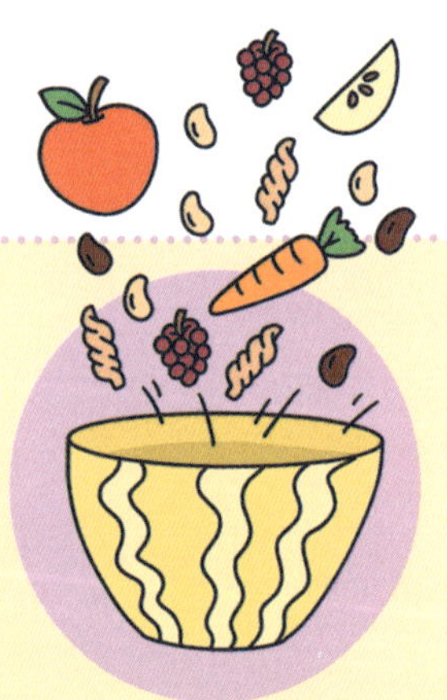

1. **Boost fibre intake:** Aim to include plenty of fibre-rich foods in your child's diet. Offer fruits with the skin on, vegetables, whole grains, beans and lentils. You can also add fibre supplements like psyllium husk if needed, but consult your doctor first.

2. **Hydrate, hydrate, hydrate:** Ensure your child drinks plenty of water and other fluids throughout the day. This helps soften poo and makes it easier to pass.

3. **Establish a toilet routine:** Encourage your child to sit on the toilet for a few minutes after meals, even if they don't feel the urge. This can help establish a regular bowel pattern.

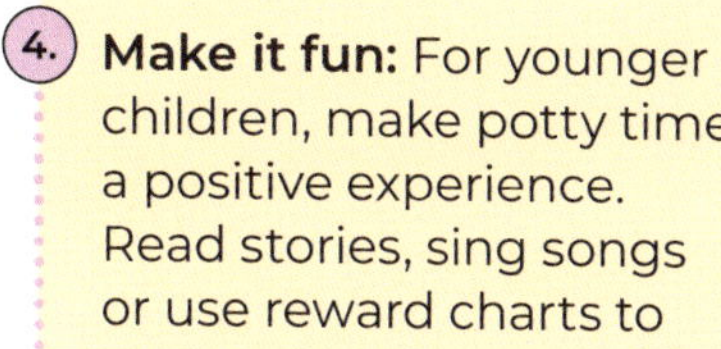

4. **Make it fun:** For younger children, make potty time a positive experience. Read stories, sing songs or use reward charts to encourage them.

5. **Over-the-counter remedies:** In consultation with your doctor, consider using stool softeners (laxatives), lubricants or suppositories for short-term relief.

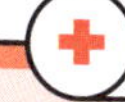

SEEK MEDICAL HELP

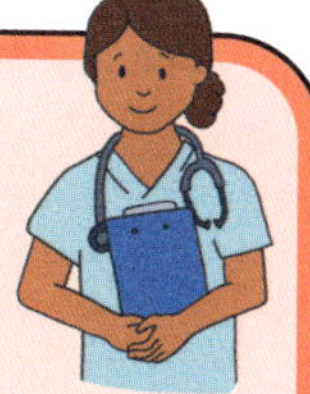

Seek medical attention if your child's constipation persists or worsens, or if they experience any of the following:

- severe abdominal pain
- blood in the stool or upon wiping
- vomiting
- unexplained weight loss
- sudden onset of constipation.

Remember: Early intervention is key. With proper guidance and support, most children can overcome constipation and establish healthy bowel habits.

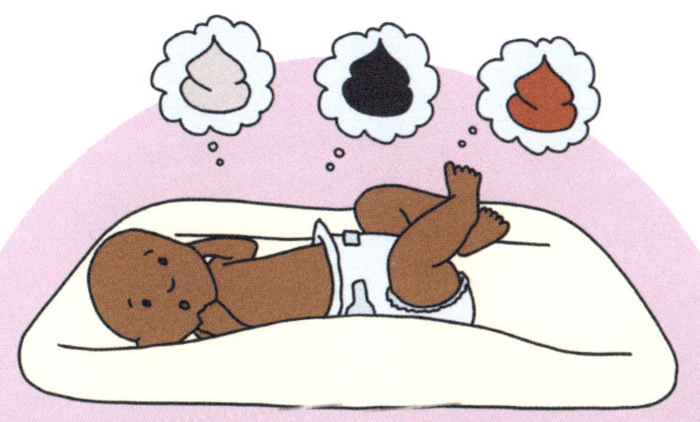

Coughing

If your child's cough is keeping you up at night, you're not alone. Coughing is one of the most common reasons parents bring their children to the doctor. Children can often enter coughing paroxysms or fits, where they start and never seem to stop, sometimes resulting in a vomit (we call this post-tussive emesis).

Why do children cough?

Coughing is a reflex that helps clear the airways of mucus, irritants or germs. It's a smart reflex! However, persistent or severe coughing can be a sign of an underlying issue.

Common causes of coughing in children:

- **Colds and respiratory infections:** The most common cause of coughing in children is an obvious one – a simple cold or other viral infection of the respiratory system.
- **Allergies:** Allergens like pollen, house dust mite or pet dander can irritate the airways and trigger coughing.
- **Asthma:** Coughing, especially at night or with exercise, can be a sign of asthma. One of the sneakiest signs of asthma (which is often missed) is a child being cough-free during the day, and suddenly having cough onset when they go to bed. This is called nocturnal cough and it responds brilliantly to simple asthma treatment.
- **Post-nasal drip:** Mucus dripping down the back of the throat can cause a tickly cough.
- **Irritants:** Second-hand smoke, pollution or even dry air can irritate the airways and lead to coughing.

When should you be concerned?

Most coughs in children are nothing to worry about and will resolve on their own.

However, you should talk to your local doctor if your child's cough:

- lasts more than two weeks
- is accompanied by difficulty breathing, wheezing or a high fever
- produces bloody or discoloured mucus
- wakes them up at night
- interferes with or limits their daily activities
- is associated with other features, like unexplained weight loss.

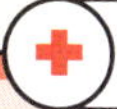

SEEK MEDICAL HELP

If you're concerned about your child's cough, don't hesitate to talk to your doctor. We can help determine the cause of the cough and recommend the most appropriate treatment.

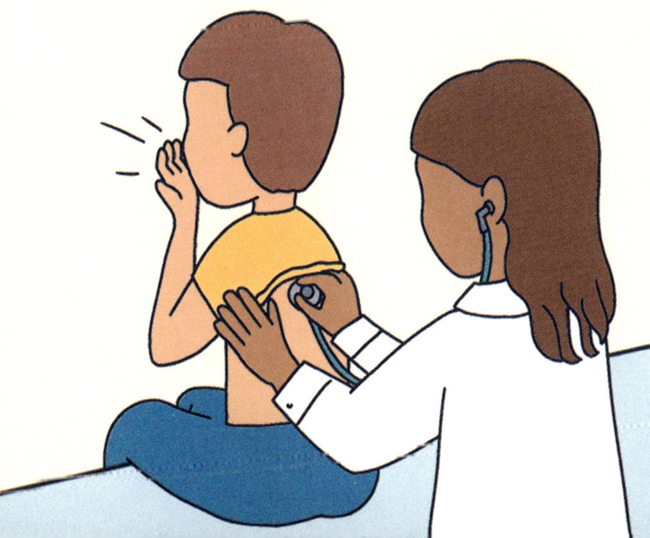

Soothing your child's cough

Here are some tips to help your child feel more comfortable:

1. **Hydration:** Encourage them to drink plenty of fluids like water, clear soup, warm tea or warm honey water.
2. **Humidifier:** A cool-mist humidifier can help moisten the air and soothe irritated airways. Aromatherapy oils are not recommended.
3. **Saline drops or spray:** These can help loosen mucus and make it easier to cough up.
4. **Elevate the head of the bed:** Slightly elevating the head of your child's bed can help reduce night-time coughing. Be mindful of safe sleep tips for younger children (this is not advised for babies).
5. **Home changes:** Consider more frequent vacuuming and linen changes to reduce pet fur and house dust mite, and close windows on high-pollen days or when neighbours are mowing the lawn.
6. **Rest:** Adequate rest is essential for the body to fight off infection.
7. **Avoid irritants:** Keep your home smoke-free and minimise exposure to other irritants like strong perfumes or cleaning products.
8. **Lubricate the throat:** this might be with an icypole (an oral hydration version will also be helpful if they are unwell) or for older children, a lozenge they can suck on. Talk to your pharmacist for a sugar-free option to protect their teeth.

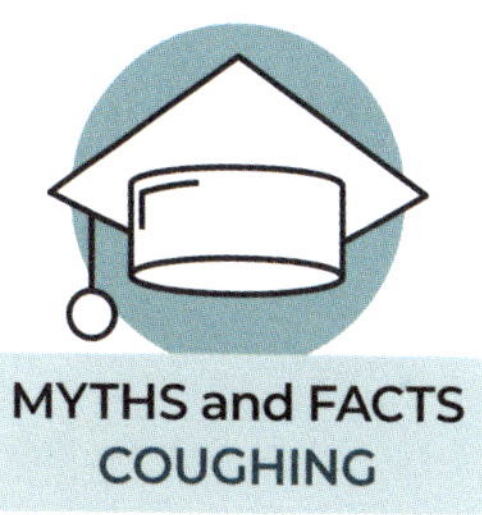

MYTHS and FACTS COUGHING

Myth: All coughs need medication.

Fact: Most coughs are caused by viruses that need to run their course. Cough suppressants are generally not recommended for young children and may even be harmful. One of their more common ingredients is codeine, which can be very constipating for some.

Myth: Honey is a miracle cure for coughs.

Fact: Honey can be soothing, but it's not recommended for children younger than twelve months due to the rare risk of botulism. While it's not a miracle cure, it can help soothe a sore throat. If your child is over twelve months I recommend a cup of warm water with a teaspoon of honey stirred through. It will be soothing and sweet and will help them stay hydrated. Remember to gently clean the teeth after a cup of honey tea.

 **Remember:**

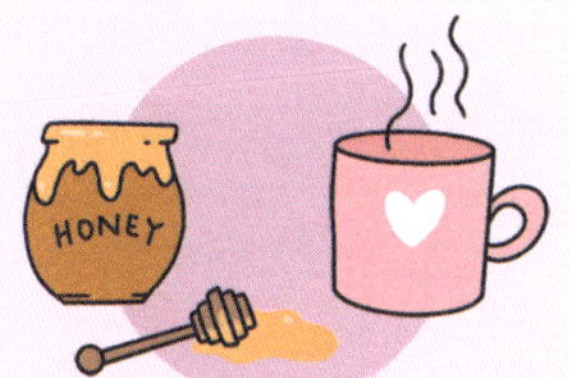

- Most coughs are harmless and will resolve on their own.
- Focus on keeping your child comfortable and hydrated.
- Don't hesitate to seek medical advice if you're concerned.

Breathing difficulties

Breathing difficulty (or increased work of breathing) is one of the key signs of severe illness in children. And it can be quite scary, as a parent, if you don't know what to look for or how to assess the work of breathing. So let's go through what you need to know.

Parents need to pay attention to any breathing red flags – where your child is breathing **harder**, **faster** or **noisier**. Any of these should prompt immediate medical attention. Another red flag is a **retraction**, which is when the area between the ribs or below the neck sucks in when a child tries to inhale. Retractions are a sign that your child is working hard to breathe.

See pg. 9

How to assess work of breathing

Undress your child: It's best to assess your child's breathing when they are completely uncovered – this will help you identify retractions.

Checking for retractions

Neck retraction:

- A tracheal tug is a visible pulling or tugging in the neck area, just above the collarbone or sternum (breastbone), which occurs when someone is having difficulty breathing.
- It's a sign of respiratory distress and indicates that the person is working harder to breathe, often seen in conditions like croup, asthma or severe respiratory infections.

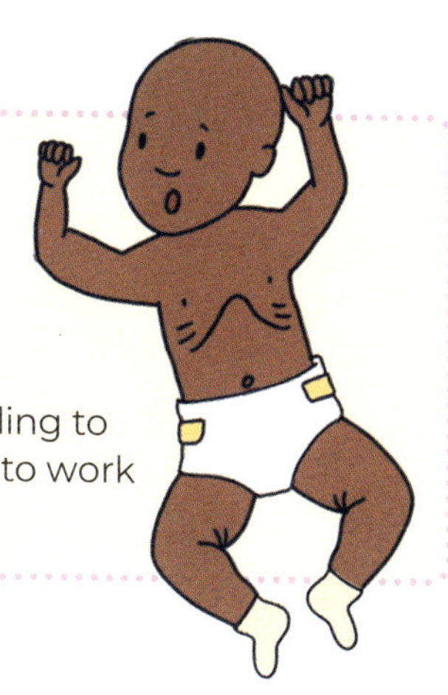

2. Rib cage retraction:

- Rib cage retractions are a sign of respiratory distress; the skin between the ribs sucks inwards during breathing.
- This occurs when someone is struggling to breathe and the chest muscles have to work extra hard to inhale air.

Signs of laboured breathing

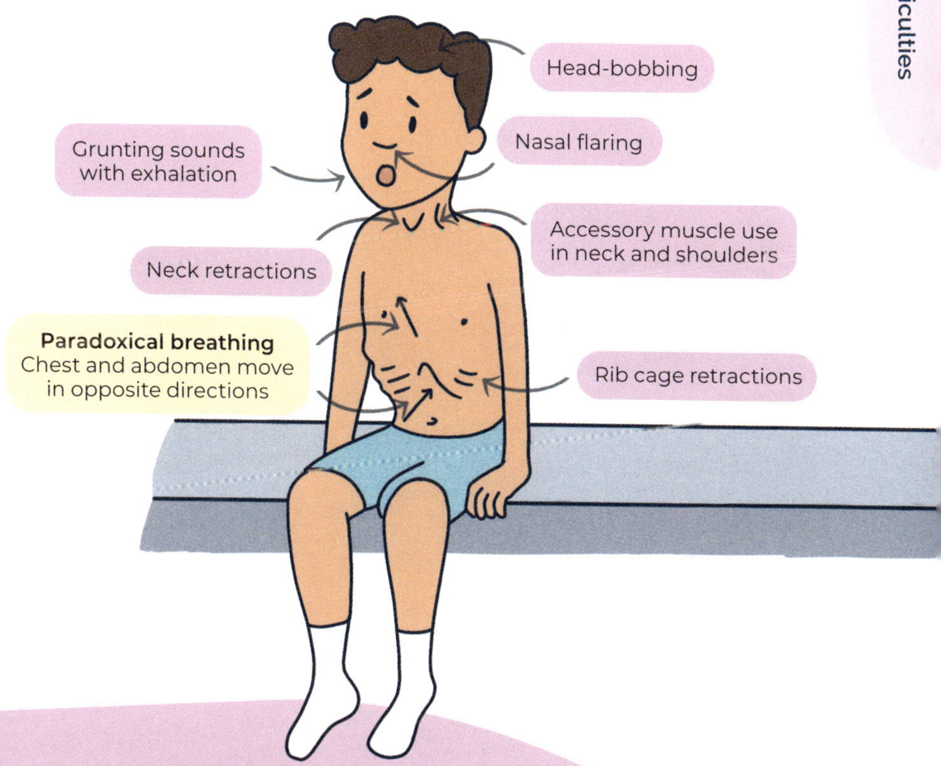

Head-bobbing
Grunting sounds with exhalation
Nasal flaring
Accessory muscle use in neck and shoulders
Neck retractions
Paradoxical breathing
Chest and abdomen move in opposite directions
Rib cage retractions

3. **Other signs of increased work of breathing:**

- Nasal flaring: the nostrils widen with each in-breath.
- Grunting: a grunt sound occurs with each out-breath.
- Head-bobbing: the head bobs up and down with each breath, a sign that the neck muscles are being used.
- Respiratory rate: rapid, shallow breathing.
- Accessory muscle use: the muscles in the neck, shoulders or abdomen are used to try to increase the lung capacity. The child may have their shoulders up and their belly out.
- Paradoxical breathing: the chest and abdomen move in opposite directions.
- Wheeze or stridor: abnormal breath sounds.
- Difficulty speaking: if the child can only speak in one- or two-word sentences.
- Pale or blue discolouration to the lips or nail beds can be a sign of low oxygen levels.

Is your baby or child breathing faster than normal?
Babies already breathe quite fast: forty breaths per minute compared to between twelve and twenty breaths per minute for adults. If your baby is taking more than sixty breaths per minute or appears be having trouble catching their breath, you should call an ambulance.

For older children and adolescents, instead of focusing on the breathing rate, try to determine whether your child is 'working hard to breathe' or gasping.

If your child displays increased work of breathing or a rapid breathing (respiratory) rate, have them seen by a doctor immediately. Breathing difficulty is one of the significant signs of illness in children and should never be ignored.

Rashes

First-aid kit items:

- a glass

Rashes can be pretty confronting, but the good news is that most of them tend to be benign.

The critical thing to know about rashes is whether they are:

- blanching, or
- non-blanching (cause for immediate concern).

How to assess if a rash is blanching:

Technique 1: Push down on the child's rash with your finger.

- If you push down on the rash and it disappears, it is a blanching rash. If the rash doesn't disappear, it is non-blanching.
- With a blanching rash, the rash will come back again very quickly when you remove your finger.

Technique 2: Push down on your child's rash with a glass.

- Press the side of the glass down on the rash so that you can see the depressed skin.
- If the rash turns skin colour beneath the glass as you press down on it, it's a blanching rash. If there is no change, it is a non-blanching rash.

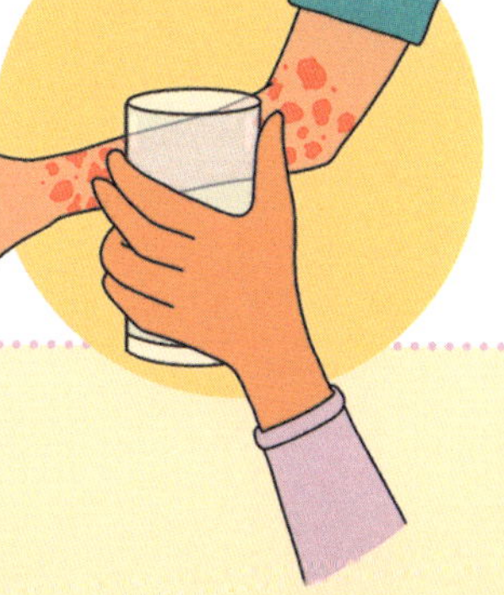

When to worry about blanching rashes (the ones that disappear):

While blanching rashes are mostly benign, there are some situations when they are a concern:

1. When they come on really quickly.
2. When they spread over the whole body (this might be an infection).
3. When they're associated with difficulty breathing (this might be an allergic rash).

Get these seen to as soon as possible.

Non-blanching rashes:

Whether you're using your finger or a glass, a non-blanching rash **will not disappear**.

- It will remain red or purple.
- It will not turn skin colour.

If your child has a non-blanching rash and a temperature, you should call triple-0 or take them to the emergency department as soon as possible.

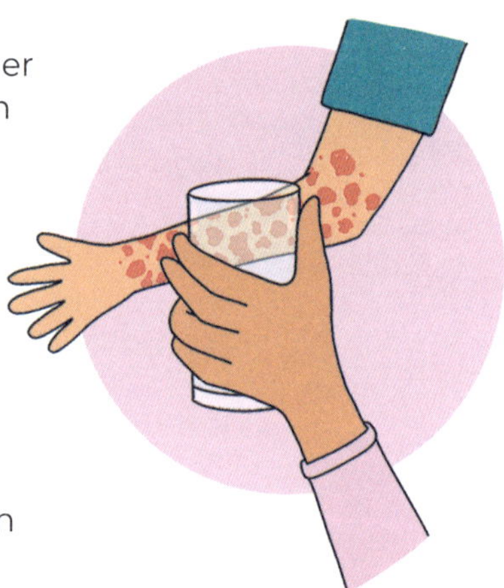

The concern here is for meningococcal disease, which can present as:

1. sepsis (page 171)
2. meningitis (page 146).

It's important that you get your child seen to immediately, as they could deteriorate very quickly.

Rashes and temperature

Be aware: does your child's rash occur with a temperature? It's not uncommon for a rash to occur at the end of a febrile illness (a fever), almost like a post-viral shedding. In this case, you will see the rash after the fever breaks and the temperature comes down.

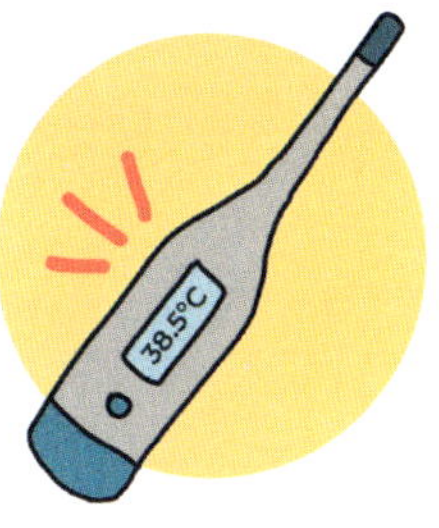

BUT if a rash occurs in association with a fever, you should always go and get it checked as soon as possible – it's considered a medical emergency.

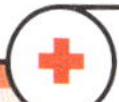

SEEK MEDICAL HELP

1. Your child is under three months of age – there is a lower threshold for dealing with temperatures in young babies.
2. The child has had a temperature for more than forty-eight hours.

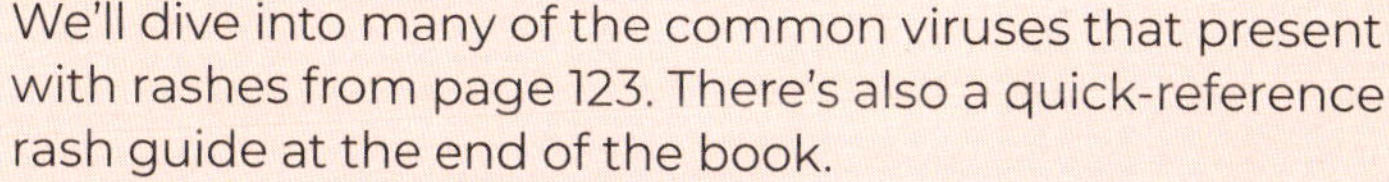

We'll dive into many of the common viruses that present with rashes from page 123. There's also a quick-reference rash guide at the end of the book.

Skin infections

Babies and young children have developing immune systems, which make them more susceptible to infections than adults. Their delicate skin can easily be broken, allowing in bacteria, viruses, fungi or parasites.

Common symptoms of skin infections:

- redness or discolouration of the skin
- a rash or bumps on the skin
- itching, pain or discomfort
- swelling or warmth in the affected area
- fever.

When to seek a medical opinion:

- if the infection rapidly spreads or worsens
- if your child has ongoing fever or appears to be in pain
- if the skin infection does not improve with basic care or over-the-counter treatments.

Prompt diagnosis and appropriate treatment are crucial for managing skin infections.

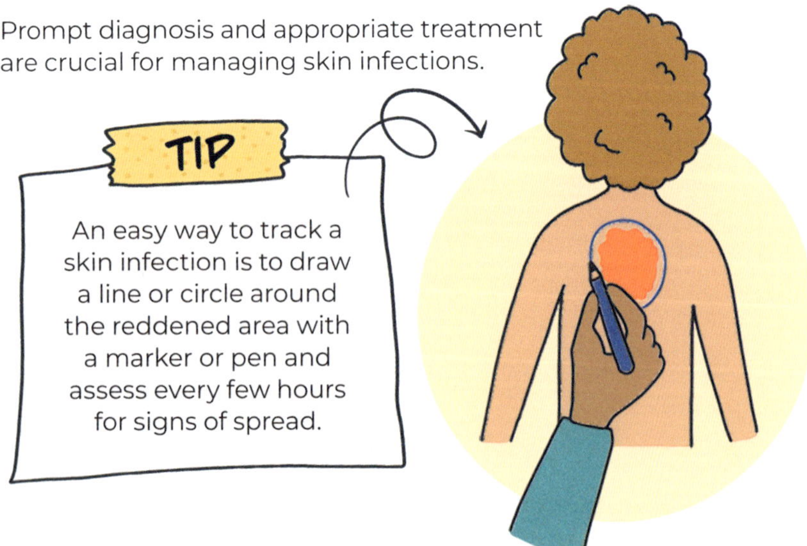

Pain and pain medication

Pain is not fun for anyone, especially children. Thankfully, there are safe and effective ways to help them feel better.

Pain is a signal that something's not right in the body.

- It can be caused by a variety of things, from a scraped knee to a stomach ache or something more sinister.
- It's important to listen to your child's pain cues and take them seriously, as they might not always be able to express exactly what they're feeling.

When it comes to pain relief for children, there are several options available, each with its own benefits and considerations.

For mild to moderate pain:

Over-the-counter medications like paracetamol or ibuprofen are often effective.

Taste matters:

Some pain medications are tolerated better than others – flavour plays a big role. If your child is refusing to take a particular brand of pain relief, consider switching to a different brand – the change in flavour may be better tolerated.

Always read the label:

It's important to follow the recommended dosage based on your child's age and weight. Some pain medications come in different concentrations so reading the label is crucial. What was 5 ml of one bottle may equate to 2.5 ml in a different concentration. Consult with your doctor or pharmacist if you have any questions.

For severe pain:

Your doctor might prescribe stronger pain medications or recommend other treatments, such as heat or cold therapy, massage or physical therapy. It's important to discuss all options with your doctor to determine the best approach for your child's specific needs.

In an emergency setting (i.e. paramedic or emergency department use), children might be given stronger medicines in controlled conditions. These might include methoxyflurane (the green stick), nasal fentanyl, ketamine or other opioids. While these medicines may frighten parents, when used in appropriate doses by healthcare professionals they are safe for and well tolerated by children.

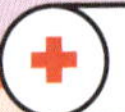

SEEK MEDICAL HELP

- If your baby is under three months of age and unwell enough to need medicine, they need to be assessed by a doctor. Don't give medication until you've talked to a doctor.
- If your child has been using pain medication for more than forty-eight hours, you need to have them reviewed by a doctor.
- If your child's pain is persistent, severe or accompanied by other symptoms like fever, vomiting or difficulty breathing, seek medical attention immediately.

Giving your child both paracetamol and ibuprofen

So that your child's pain is well controlled, it is OK to alternate doses of paracetamol and ibuprofen, or even to give both at the same time. Spacing doses out means that your child can receive pain relief frequently throughout the day. Remember to follow the dosing guide and do not exceed the recommended frequency per day – see notes on tracking medication on page 45.

	Paracetamol	Ibuprofen
Popular brands	Panadol, Panamax, Dymadon and Tylenol	Nurofen, Brufen and Advil
How much do I give?	Always give the dose that is written on the bottle or packet according to your child's age and weight.	Always give the dose that is written on the bottle or packet according to your child's age and weight.
How frequently can I give it?	Doses can be given every four to six hours – but no more than **four** times in twenty-four hours.	Doses can be given every six to eight hours, but no more than **three** times in twenty-four hours.
Complications?	Paracetamol can be dangerous in overdose or with prolonged use.	There are rare but serious side effects if ibuprofen is given to a child for a prolonged time.
Does it upset the stomach?	No.	Short-term use of ibuprofen, at appropriate doses, may be taken with a glass of water and no food. If this causes stomach upset, try offering your child some food or milk.
When to seek help	If you need to give your child paracetamol for more than forty-eight hours, you should take them to see a doctor.	If you need to give your child ibuprofen for more than forty-eight hours, you should take them to see a doctor.

Many common cold and flu formulations contain either paracetamol or ibuprofen. Be careful not to 'double dose' if using a combination treatment.

Don't give aspirin to children under twelve years of age, unless directly advised by your doctor.

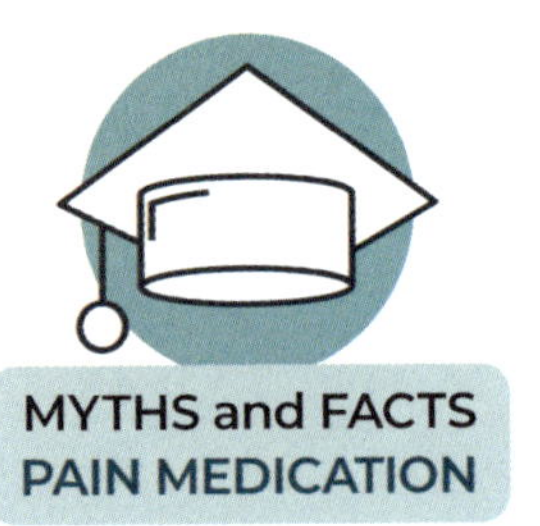

Myth: Children have to eat if you give them ibuprofen or they'll get a stomach ulcer.

Fact: When used in high doses for long periods of time, ibuprofen can prompt stomach issues, but infrequent doses can certainly be given on an empty stomach. You do not need to force food or milk when giving your child ibuprofen.

Myth: You can't use paracetamol and ibuprofen together.

Fact: Always read the label of any medication you are using, but paracetamol and ibuprofen can be used together, because they have different mechanisms of action. If your child needs this much pain relief, you might want to see your local doctor to be sure.

Myth: You can't give pain medication to a child under three months.

Fact: You can give pain medication to a young baby, but you should always check with your doctor first.

What's the risk of giving too much pain medication?

Giving a child an incorrect dose or giving doses of pain medication too frequently can have serious side effects. Too much paracetamol can harm your child's liver and sometimes their kidneys. Too much ibuprofen can cause stomach upsets, or sometimes it can impact breathing and make a person very drowsy.

If your child has had too much paracetamol or ibuprofen, call the Poisons Information Centre (13 11 26 in Australia) or take them to the nearest hospital emergency department.

Certain medicines should never be used in children with specific medical conditions or allergies. Never give medicine to a child in your care before checking with their parent or guardian, as even 'safe and simple' medicines can be harmful.

Tracking when you give pain medication is really important

If your child is sick, it's almost certain that you – and they – are sleep deprived. And, if you have more than one child sick and more than one type of medication, it's very easy to become confused. It doesn't have to be complicated, though – keep a notepad next to the medicine, document doses in text messages with your partner or print out my illness tracker on page 45.

What to note

Medication:

- when you gave the medication
- how much was given
- which type was given.

Your child's temperature:

- Remember, don't focus on the exact number – just the trend over time.

See pg. 12

Hydration:

- fluid in
- fluid out (nappies or toilet trips).

Any other symptoms:

Other symptoms worth noting down might include nausea, loss of appetite, headache or anything else unusual.

Taking these simple notes will help you and other carers keep track of what's happening even when you're all exhausted. If the illness progresses, this tracker will also be a very valuable source of information for your healthcare provider.

Pain relief isn't just about medication

There are many non-pharmaceutical ways to help your child feel better, too:

- cuddles
- distraction techniques like reading a book or watching a movie
- ice packs or cool face washers
- coloured Band-Aids with their favourite character
- soothing rehydration ice blocks
- even just a calming presence can go a long way in reducing pain and anxiety.

As a parent, you know your child best. Trust your instincts and advocate for your child's wellbeing. With the right support and a little TLC, you can help your little one overcome pain and get back to their happy, playful self.

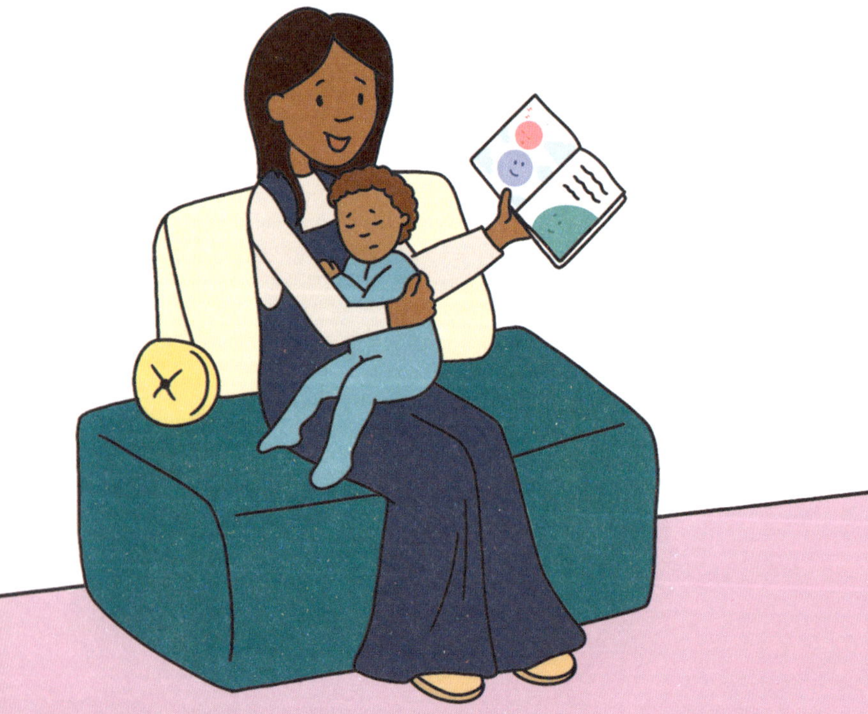

EXAMPLE

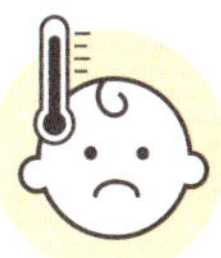

Illness tracker

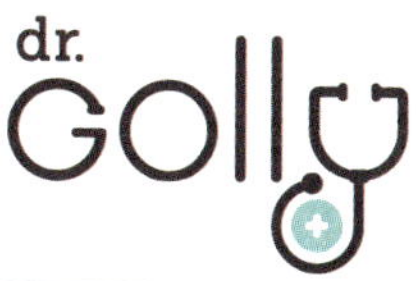

Name: *Jack* Age: *3* Date: *12/02*

Signs & symptoms:

- *Lethargic and flat*
- *Runny poo*
-
-

Temperature:

Time	Temperature
6.30am	*38.1* °C / °F
	°C / °F
	°C / °F
	°C / °F
	°C / °F

Nappies or toilet:

Time	Wee	Poo	Vomit
3am			✓
6am	✓		
7am			✓

Medication:

Time	Type	Dosage
6.35am	*paracetamol*	*3.5 ml*

PARACETAMOL: MAX. DOSES 4 IN 24 HRS
IBUPROFEN: MAX. DOSES 3 IN 24 HRS

... read instructions on medication carefully and ... directed. If symptoms persist, please consult a ... professional.

Fluid intake:

Time	Type	Amount
3.30am	*water*	*50 ml*

...s/notes:

Scan here
to download your printable illness tracker

Viral vs bacterial infections

If your child has a fever, cough, runny nose or upset tummy, you're probably wondering: *is it just a virus or something more serious, like a bacterial infection?* As a father and paediatrician, I understand the concern – it's a question I ask almost every day.

It can be challenging to tell viral and bacterial infections apart, but knowing the key differences can help you understand your child's illness and the best course of action, especially the importance of avoiding unnecessary antibiotics.

Let's delve into the world of viruses and bacteria to understand how they affect our little ones.

Tiny troublemakers: viruses vs bacteria
Both viruses and bacteria are tiny germs that can cause infections, but they're quite different creatures.

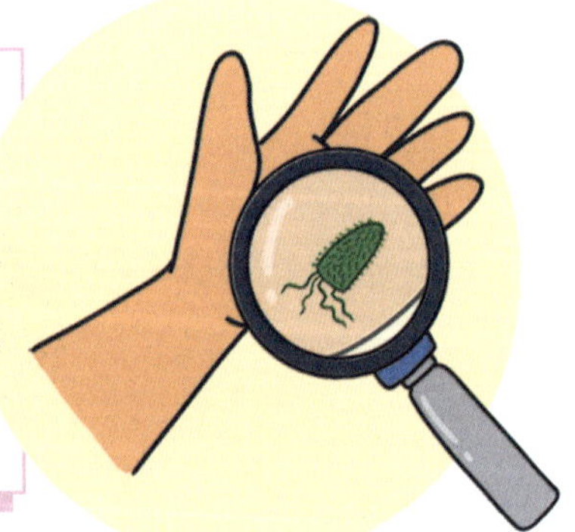

	Viruses	Bacteria
	20-200 nanometre	1,000 nanometre
Size	Extremely small, can only be seen with a powerful microscope.	Larger than viruses; some can be seen with a regular microscope.
Structure	Simple structure, basically genetic material inside a protein coat.	More complex structure, with cell walls and organelles.
How they work	Viruses invade healthy cells and use them to reproduce.	Bacteria multiply on their own, sometimes producing toxins that make us sick.
Common illnesses caused	Colds, flu, gastroenteritis, chickenpox, measles, most sore throats, bronchiolitis.	Strep throat, ear infections, some sinus infections, urinary tract infections (UTIs), pneumonia.
Treatment	Usually, the body's immune system fights off viral infections on its own. Some antiviral medications are available for specific viruses.	Antibiotics are often used to treat bacterial infections.

Decoding your child's symptoms

While viral and bacterial infections can cause similar symptoms, there are some clues that might help you distinguish between them:

1. **Fever:** High fevers (above 39°C) are more common with bacterial infections, though this is not always the case.
2. **Onset:** Viral infections often start gradually, while bacterial infections (see page 46) may begin and progress more rapidly.
3. **Mucus:** Thick, green or yellow mucus might suggest a bacterial infection, but this is not a universal rule.
4. **Duration:** Viral infections typically last a few days to a week, while bacterial infections may linger or worsen without treatment.

Bacteria vs virus

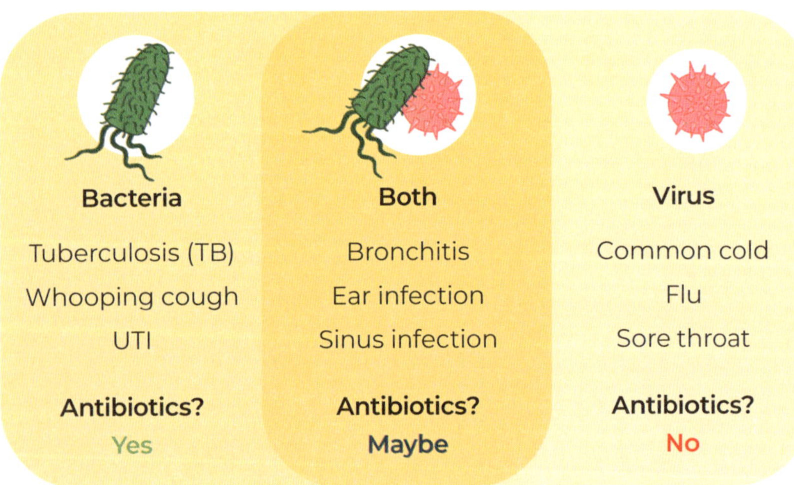

Specific symptoms: Some symptoms are more suggestive of one type of infection than the other. For example, a urinary tract infection (UTI; see page 186) is more likely to be bacterial, while a cough with a runny nose is more often viral.

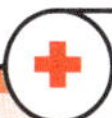

SEEK MEDICAL HELP

It's not always easy to tell the difference between viral and bacterial infections based on symptoms alone. If you're unsure or if your child seems very unwell, it's always best to consult your doctor. We can perform tests, like a throat swab or urine test, to determine if a bacterial infection is present and needs antibiotics.

MYTHS and FACTS VIRUSES VS BACTERIA

Myth: Antibiotics cure everything.

Fact: Antibiotics only work against bacterial infections. They have no effect on viruses. Giving antibiotics unnecessarily not only results in gastrointestinal changes, it negatively impacts the gut microbiome (ecosystem of good and bad bacteria that play an important role in digestion as well as overall health and wellbeing). It also increases antibiotic resistance, a problem for everyone in the community.

Myth: Green or yellow mucus always means it's a bacterial infection.

Fact: Mucus colour can change during the course of a viral infection. Coloured mucus can also occur in viruses, or in the setting of inflammation. It's not a reliable indicator of whether antibiotics are needed. Red or dark brown phlegm may indicate bleeding in the airway and should be reviewed by a doctor. It's helpful to take a photo of the phlegm to show your child's doctor.

Myth: It's always better to be safe and take antibiotics.

Fact: Overuse of antibiotics can lead to antibiotic resistance, making them less effective when we really need them.

A note on secondary infections

Sometimes, a viral infection becomes complicated by a secondary bacterial infection. If your child has a virus and seems to be improving but suddenly becomes more unwell, this may signal a bacterial complication, which could require antibiotics. Discuss this with your child's doctor, as the original situation has now changed.

Supporting your child's recovery

Whether it's a viral or bacterial infection, here are some tips to help your child feel better:

Rest:

Encourage plenty of rest to help their body fight off the infection.

Hydration:

Make sure they drink plenty of fluids to prevent dehydration.

Symptom relief:

Use over-the-counter medications (as directed) to relieve fever, aches and pains.

Hygiene:

Teach your child to wash their hands frequently and cover their coughs and sneezes to prevent spreading germs.

 **Remember:**

Trust your instincts: If you're worried about your child, don't hesitate to seek medical advice.

Ask questions: Don't be afraid to ask your doctor for clarification if you're unsure about the course.

By understanding the differences between viral and bacterial infections, you'll be better equipped to navigate your child's illnesses and advocate for their health.

Immunisation schedule

As a father and a paediatrician, one of my biggest joys is seeing kids grow up healthy and strong. A huge part of achieving this is through childhood immunisation – a topic that's sometimes met with questions and concerns.

Let's unravel this aspect of your child's health journey together, covering everything from the basics to the finer details, debunking myths and empowering you with knowledge to make the best decisions for your little one.

Why immunisation is your child's best defence

Immunisation, often called vaccination, is like giving your child a superhero shield against some of the nastiest villains in the disease world. These villains, like measles, whooping cough (pertussis) and polio pneumococcus (to name just a few), were once major threats to children's health. Thankfully, vaccines have drastically reduced their impact, but they haven't disappeared entirely, which is why immunisation remains crucial.

How do vaccines work?

Vaccines most commonly work by introducing a weakened or inactive form of a virus or bacteria to your child's body. This 'sneak peek' or 'warning shot' allows their immune system to build up a memory of the invader, so if they ever encounter the real thing, their body is ready to fight back swiftly and effectively.

The National Immunisation Program (NIP): Australia's shield of protection

The Australian government understands the importance of protecting children, which is why it provides free vaccines for all children under the National Immunisation Program (NIP). This comprehensive program covers a wide range of diseases and is regularly updated based on the latest scientific evidence and population data to ensure your child receives the most effective protection.

You can find the complete NIP schedule on the Australian Department of Health website, outlining which vaccines are recommended at different ages. It is worth referring to this every few months, to monitor for any changes to the schedule that may impact your children. The program is designed to provide optimal protection at key developmental stages, from infancy through to adolescence. Some children are eligible for extra vaccines, depending on their health status and cultural background.

Remember, though, the NIP is not a complete list of vaccines available to your child. For example, while the NIP includes the MenACWY (meningococcal A, C, W and Y) vaccination for all children at twelve months, this vaccination – as well as the Bexsero (meningococcal B) vaccination – can be safely administered from six weeks of age at a cost to parents. This provides protection against meningococcal disease during infancy, one of the most vulnerable times. BCG vaccine against tuberculosis (TB) is another optional vaccine (see travel vaccinations on page 56). It is worth further discussing these with your vaccination provider.

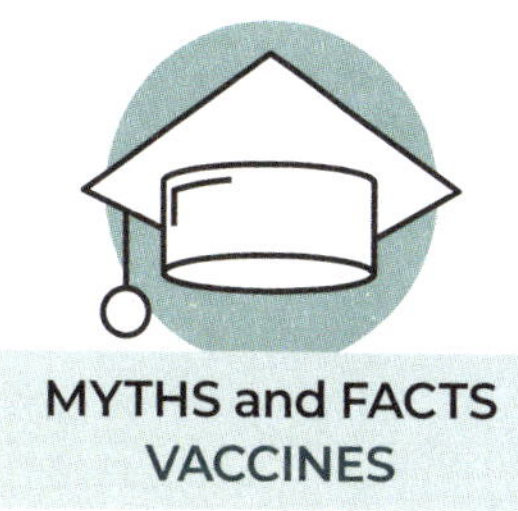

MYTHS and FACTS VACCINES

Myth: Vaccines are not safe.

Fact: Vaccines undergo rigorous testing and are among the safest and most effective medical interventions available. Serious side effects are incredibly rare.

Myth: Vaccines cause autism.

Fact: There is no scientific evidence linking vaccines to autism. This myth has been thoroughly debunked by numerous studies, but remains a stubborn thorn.

Myth: Natural immunity is better than vaccine-acquired immunity.

Fact: While natural immunity can be protective, it often comes at a cost: experiencing a potentially severe illness. Vaccines provide a safe and controlled way to build immunity without risk of the disease or its complications. Chickenpox is a terrific example of this – parents used to arrange 'chickenpox parties' to intentionally expose their child and cause infection, hoping to speed up natural immunity. Thankfully, vaccines have put an end to these events!

Your questions, answered

It's natural for parents to have questions about vaccines. Here are some common ones I hear in my practice:

Why does my child need so many vaccines?

Each vaccine targets a specific disease, and the timing is carefully designed to maximise protection when your child is most vulnerable. Vaccines also have a cumulative effect, and several doses may be required to achieve the best protection.

Can vaccines overload my child's immune system?

No. Children's immune systems are exposed to countless germs every day. Vaccines are designed to work with their immune system, not overwhelm it.

My child is healthy – do they really need all these vaccines?

Yes! Vaccines protect even the healthiest children from potentially serious illnesses. Don't forget that immunising a child also creates a cocoon of protection for your entire family, so bugs are less likely to circulate through to other family members, including the elderly (this is called herd protection).

What about side effects?

Most side effects from vaccines are mild and temporary, like a sore arm or low-grade fever. Serious reactions are very rare.

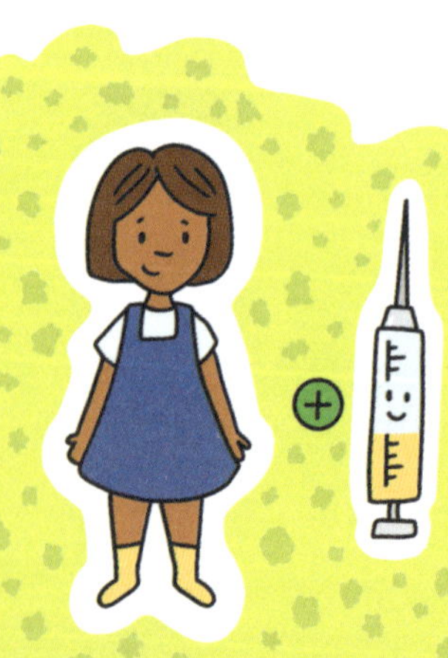

Your partner in your child's health journey

As a paediatrician, I believe that knowledge is empowering. I encourage you to have open and honest conversations with your doctor or paediatrician about any questions or concerns you have regarding vaccines. We're here to provide you with accurate information and support you in making informed decisions for your child's health.

Remember, every vaccine your child receives is a step towards a healthier future. By choosing to vaccinate, you're not only protecting your child but also contributing to the health and wellbeing of our entire community.

We're on the same team

One of my favourite roles as a paediatrician was in the immunisation clinic of the Royal Children's Hospital in Melbourne. This specialised clinic was formed to give vaccine-hesitant parents the opportunity to raise their concerns, discuss their child's previous reactions and have open discussions about the risks and benefits of vaccines. Each shift, I met parents who were shocked to find that I was not there to fight with them. The most important thing to understand about vaccines is that doctors and parents are members of the SAME team, with a singular focus on the best outcome for the child. We all want the same thing – what is best for the child. If you are nervous or hesitant about vaccines, or have read or heard something concerning, you should absolutely discuss it with your child's doctor. I will always have non-judgemental discussions about vaccines, the diseases they prevent and the side-effects involved. I will present scientific data and dispel myths that circulate on the internet. If you make the considered decision not to vaccinate your child, I will not judge you or criticise you. Rather, I will further empower you to manage illnesses as they arrive and continue to support your family in our shared goal of the best possible future for your child.

Travel immunisations

It's exciting to dream about new sights, sounds and experiences. If you're planning a family adventure overseas, I want to remind you of one crucial aspect of trip preparation: travel immunisations. It is essential you ensure your child is up to date on their vaccinations and that they receive any recommended ones for your destination. And it is worth considering additional vaccinations depending on your destination – for personalised advice, it is best to see a family travel clinic.

While Australia boasts a high standard of healthcare and a robust vaccination program, the same may not be true for every corner of the world. Different countries have different disease risks, and some illnesses that are rare or well controlled here might be more common elsewhere. One also can't rely on herd immunity when travelling.

Why travel immunisations are crucial

1. **Disease prevention:** Vaccines protect your child from serious illnesses like measles, tuberculosis (TB), yellow fever, typhoid, hepatitis A and more, which might be prevalent in your destination.

2. **Peace of mind:** Knowing your child is protected allows you to relax and enjoy your trip without constantly worrying about their health.

3. **Requirement for entry:** Some countries require proof of certain vaccinations for entry, so it's important to plan ahead. It's also important to consider the timing of vaccinations, as some may take weeks to take effect, and others might need multiple doses to achieve protection; discuss this with your doctor.

Travel immunisations: what your child needs

The specific vaccines your child needs will depend on several factors, including:

Age:

Some vaccines are recommended for specific age groups.

Destination:

The diseases prevalent in different countries vary.

Length of stay:

Longer trips might require additional protection.

Activities:

Certain activities, like hiking or visiting rural areas, might increase exposure risk.

Health conditions:

Some underlying health conditions might require additional or different vaccines.

A word on influenza:

Interestingly, the single most common infection to disrupt holidays is influenza. This is thought to be from a combination of sleep disruption, body stress from new foods and environments, and greater exposure to the virus from closer proximity in airports and during transport. Children can receive the influenza vaccine from six months of age but require two doses (one month apart) in their first year of being vaccinated. Remember, even if it's not influenza season in your home country, it might be widespread at your destination.

Here are some vaccines that might be recommended for travel, depending on your destination (there are others):

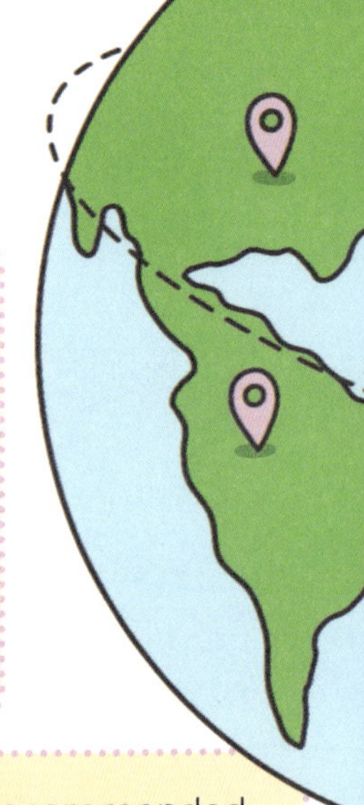

1. **Routine childhood vaccinations:** Make sure your child is up to date on the routine vaccines included in Australia's National Immunisation Program.

   It is possible to access an early, additional MMR vaccination for children between six to twelve months if travelling overseas.

2. **Hepatitis A:** Recommended for most travellers to developing countries.

3. **Typhoid:** Recommended for travellers to areas with poor sanitation.

4. **Yellow fever:** Required for entry into some countries.

5. **Japanese encephalitis:** Recommended for travellers spending extended periods in rural areas of certain Asian countries.

6. **Rabies:** Recommended for travellers who may have contact with wild animals in high-risk areas.

7. **Tuberculosis (TB):** A BCG vaccination protects against TB and is recommended for any child under five years of age (this age group is at highest risk of severe disease) travelling to a country where TB is endemic (occurs regularly). It should also be considered in a child with regular, especially longer-term, visitors in the form of family or friends from TB-endemic countries. This is a live vaccine and often needs to be organised far in advance of travelling for optimal effectiveness.

When to start planning

It's ideal to start planning your child's travel immunisations at least eight weeks before your trip. This allows enough time for the vaccines to take effect and for any follow-up doses.

Your trusted travel health adviser

The best way to determine exactly what your child needs is to consult with your local doctor or travel health clinic. They'll assess your child's individual risk factors and recommend the most appropriate vaccines for your specific itinerary.

Remember:

- **Plan ahead:** Don't leave vaccinations to the last minute.
- **Keep records:** Ensure you have a record of your child's vaccinations to show upon entry to certain countries.
- **Pack smart:** Bring along any necessary medications, insect repellent, protective clothing and sunscreen.
- **Stay informed:** Check for travel advisories and updates on disease outbreaks in your destination.
- **Organise travel insurance:** To maximise protection in the event of an unexpected illness, injury or other travel mishap, ensure your travel insurance covers all family members.

By taking the necessary precautions and ensuring your child is adequately protected, you can head off on your travels with peace of mind, knowing you've done everything you can to keep them healthy and safe. Bon voyage!

Seasonal flu and COVID-19 vaccinations

When the weather cools down and we all start reaching for our heaters again, coughs, sniffles and fevers seem to be everywhere. It can be tough to tell, though, if it's just a cold, influenza (flu) or even COVID-19. Here's the lowdown on how to tell these illnesses apart, why vaccination is so helpful, and how to keep those sniffles at bay.

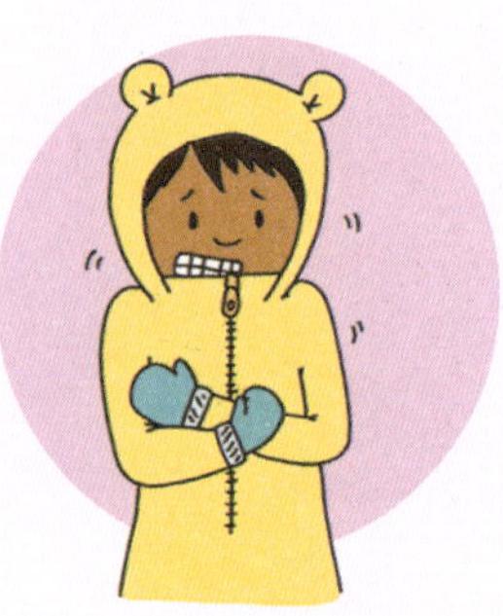

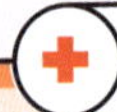

SEEK MEDICAL HELP

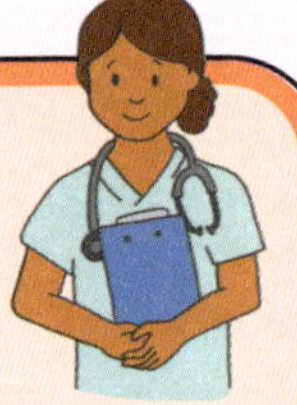

If your child shows any of these symptoms, don't wait – get them checked out right away:

- struggling to breathe
- pale or blue lips or face
- chest pain or pressure
- acting confused
- throwing up a lot or being unable to keep anything down
- signs of dehydration (dry mouth, no tears, not urinating much).

Is it the flu or COVID-19?

The flu and COVID-19 can seem pretty similar at first glance, but there are some key differences to keep in mind.

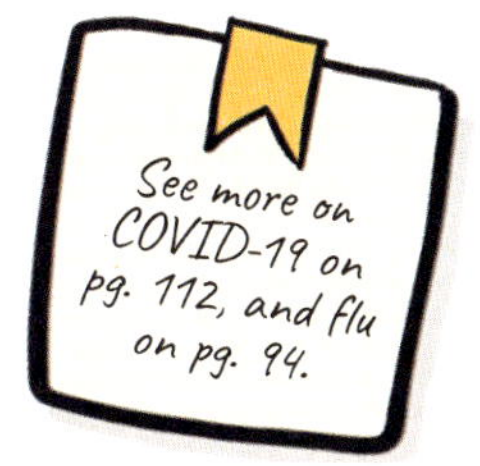

	Flu	COVID-19
Cause	Influenza viruses (multiple strains – they're sneaky!)	SARS-CoV-2 virus
Symptoms	The usual suspects: fever, cough, sore throat, runny or stuffy nose, body aches, feeling wiped out, and sometimes even an upset tummy.	Pretty much the same as the flu, but some kids also lose their sense of taste or smell, have shortness of breath, or get a rash.
Severity	Usually, it's not too bad for kids, but little ones, older folks and those with other health issues can get hit harder.	It can range from mild to severe and, sadly, there's the risk of long-term problems.
Transmission	Mostly spread through those pesky coughs and sneezes we all know too well.	Same as the flu, but it can also hang in the air longer, making it a bit trickier to avoid.
Complications	Things like pneumonia, ear infections and sinus infections are common.	Same as the flu, but kids can also get something called MIS-C (rare but serious) or have lingering symptoms (long COVID).

Vaccines: your secret weapon

Here's the great news: we've got vaccines to protect against both the flu and COVID-19. These vaccines are safe and are recommended for kids six months and older.

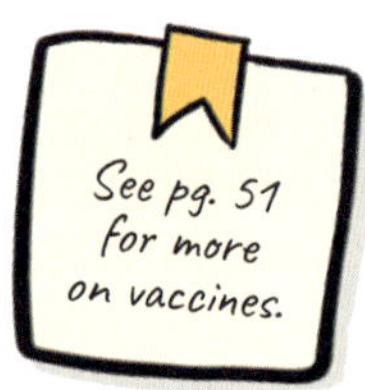

1. **Flu vaccine:** It's like a yearly tune-up for your child's immune system. The vaccine gets updated every year to match the flu strains going around, and you can usually get it from April onwards. It's especially important for little ones, kids with ongoing health problems, those planning to travel and pregnant women. All children aged six months to under five years are eligible on the NIP, and it can be purchased for older children and adults.

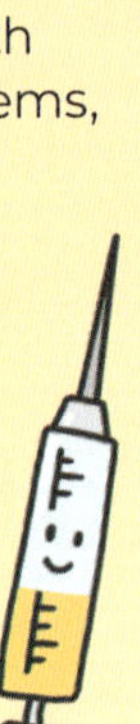

2. **COVID-19 vaccine:** This is still an evolving space, and it is best to refer to your current local recommendations. In Australia, the immunisation handbook can be accessed online. At the time of publication of this book, guidelines recommend COVID-19 primary course vaccinations for children older than six months with risk factors or severe immunocompromise. Boosters are only recommended for children with severe immunocompromise above five years of age.

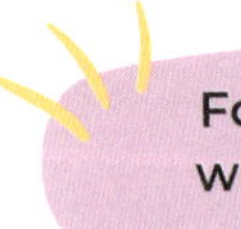

For more info, chat with your doctor or paediatrician.

More tips to keep the bugs at bay

Besides vaccines, here are some extra things you can do:

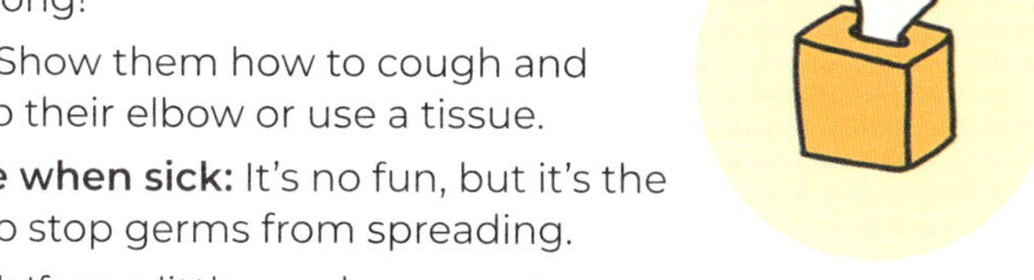

1. **Handwashing:** Teach your kids to wash their hands often with soap and water – make it a fun sing-along!
2. **Cover up:** Show them how to cough and sneeze into their elbow or use a tissue.
3. **Stay home when sick:** It's no fun, but it's the best way to stop germs from spreading.
4. **Get tested:** If your little one has symptoms, get them tested for both the flu and COVID-19 to figure out the best way to help them and prevent further spread. Home-testing kits are readily available from your local pharmacy.

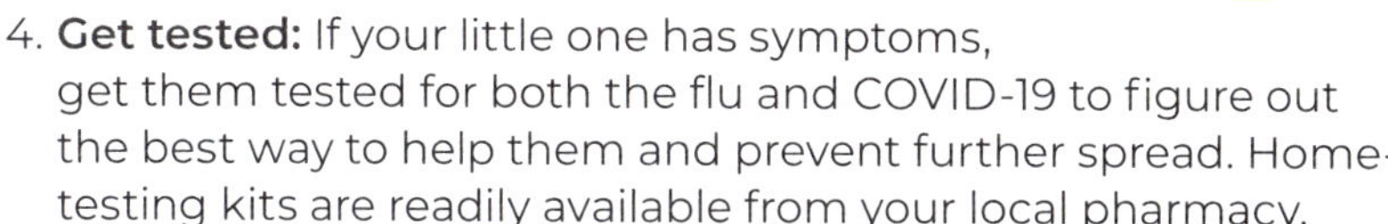

Never underestimate the importance of quality sleep to prevent illness and speed up recovery from sickness.

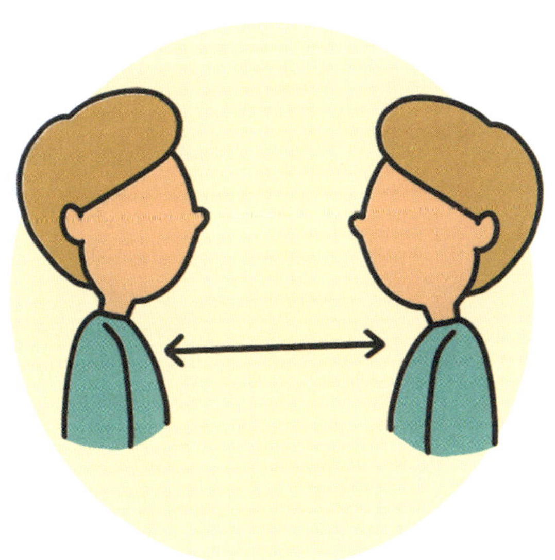

Boosting your immune system

One of the most common questions I get as a paediatrician is:

> What can I do to boost my child's immune system?

And it is usually quickly followed by:

> Should I be giving them supplements?

Boosting your child's immune system is very much about getting back to basics:

1. **Eat a balanced diet:**
    - lots of vegetables, fruit, unprocessed wholefoods and good fats
    - less sugar and highly processed food
    - for older babies and younger toddlers, make sure there's a food–milk balance.

2. **Stay hydrated:**
    - water is your best friend (make sure their drink bottle is cleaned regularly – you'd be surprised at the amount of mould and bacteria found in drink bottles)
    - minimise any juices and sugary carbonated drinks
    - caffeinated drinks should be avoided completely
    - oral rehydration solutions can be used for rapid rehydration.

3. **Get plenty of sleep :**
    - sleep is essential for all areas of development, health maintenance and disease minimisation
    - the amount of sleep a child needs varies by age (from twelve to sixteen hours a day for infants, to eight to ten hours for teenagers)
    - if your child isn't getting enough sleep, you might like to try my sleep programs.

4. **Stay active and minimise sedentary behaviour:**
   - Kids should be active for at least an hour a day, minimum – this can be formal sports or simply going for a bike ride or playing at the playground.
   - Screen time should be limited. The advice changes based on age – zero screen time for under two and no more than an hour a day for ages two to five.

5. **Manage stress:**
   - stress can make your child more prone to infection
   - allow time for whatever sparks joy
   - spend time together as a family and create opportunities for your child to explain what might be worrying them
   - if you are ever concerned by your child's emotional health, talk to your doctor.

6. **Be up to date with vaccines:**
   - see page 51.

7. **Maintain hand hygiene:**
   - This is the key! Encourage effective handwashing after using the bathroom, before eating and after touching a snotty nose or sticking a hand in their mouth.
   - Teach your child to wash and dry their hands effectively, and create gentle routines around hand hygiene.

Supplements:
If your family is focused on the seven items above, you probably don't need any additional supplements. If you think your child may benefit from a supplement, talk to your paediatrician or local doctor. Complementary and alternative therapies can also provide 'boosts' to your child's immune system.

Handwashing and hygiene

The only thing worse than having a sick baby or child is having multiple sick children – or being sick yourself as you're trying to care for your kids. When an illness enters the house, particularly a viral illness, further spread between household members is common, but you can minimise the spread with the correct hygiene practices.

Handwashing is your first line of defence for the whole family. Get everyone into the habit of washing hands before and after:

- preparing or eating food
- breastfeeding
- feeding a child
- touching, cuddling or holding a sick child
- wiping your nose or your child's nose
- giving medication or applying ointment to sores
- touching cutlery, drinking cups and other objects a sick child has touched
- changing a nappy
- using the toilet or helping a child to use the toilet
- touching a wound
- touching pets or other animals.

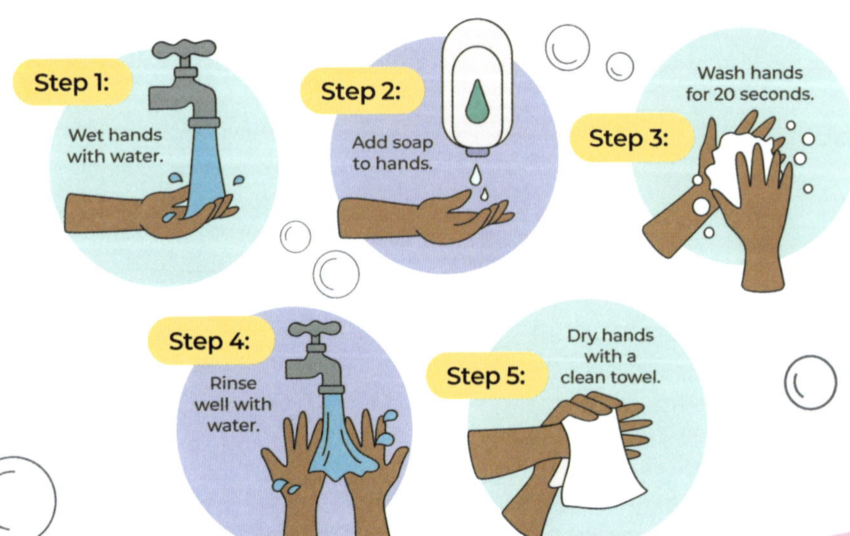

Other hygiene tips:

TIP 1:
Carry some hand sanitiser with you and use it whenever you need to decontaminate your hands. It will not work if your hands are visibly dirty, but it's a good option if you don't have hot, soapy water.

TIP 2:
Cough or sneeze into a tissue or your elbow instead of into your hands. Teach your kids to do this too.

TIP 3:
Use tissues rather than handkerchiefs.

TIP 3:
Wear disposable gloves before handling dirty nappies, or cleaning up blood or any other body fluid.

TIP 4:
When using cloth towels to dry your hands, hang the towel up to dry after each use, and launder the towels regularly. Launder bedding in hot water and detergent as required.

TIP 5:
If you suspect vomit or diarrhoea is gastro-related, put on gloves and masks when changing nappies or helping your child. Use paper towel to wipe up.

TIP 6:
If there's illness in the house, regularly clean surfaces with hot, soapy water followed by a bleach-based disinfectant. This means kitchen countertops, bathroom surfaces, toilet seats and flush handles, floors, doorknobs, and light switches. Follow all the safety packaging guidelines for bleach solutions – if not used correctly, bleach is highly toxic.

TIP 7:
Dispose of contaminated tissues, paper towel, vomit or diarrhoea in sealed bags.

TIP 8:
If one child is sick, bathe the sick child separately.

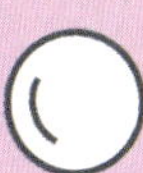
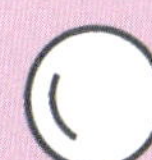

"This is a game many families are forced to play ... and no one wants to win!"

Childcare BINGO!

Some of the fun things your kids may bring home

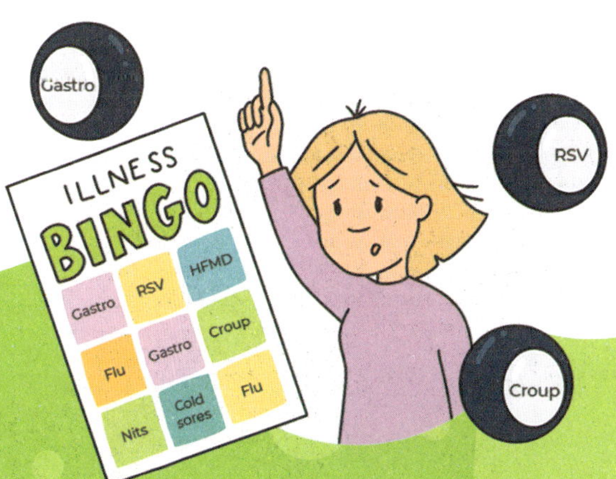

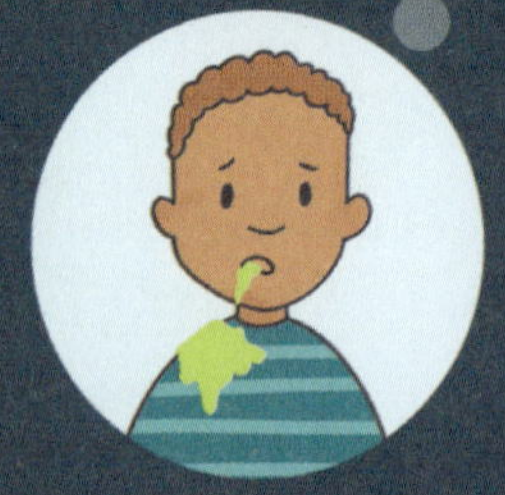

Gastrointestinal illness

Gastro pg. 71

Gastrointestinal illness

Gastro

Gastroenteritis, often called gastro or the stomach flu, is a common and rather unpleasant illness that can affect children of all ages, leaving them feeling queasy and uncomfortable.

SYMPTOMS: VOMITING, DIARRHOEA

The key is not to panic. Most cases are mild and resolve on their own with a little TLC and rehydration at home. Let's dive in and learn more about this tummy bug so you can be prepared.

What is gastroenteritis?

Gastroenteritis is an inflammation of the stomach and intestines, often caused by viruses, bacteria or parasites. It's a highly contagious illness that spreads easily through contaminated food or water, or through close contact with an infected person. Children are particularly susceptible because their immune systems are still developing, and they often have less-than-perfect hygiene habits.

When caused by a bug, gastro is referred to as infectious gastroenteritis; there is nothing quite as challenging as caring for a child with gastro while experiencing gastro yourself, so prioritise impeccable hand hygiene! Non-infectious gastro can be caused by spoiled food, food allergies, medications or underlying medical conditions, and cannot be spread from one person to another.

Common causes of infectious gastroenteritis

Viruses	Bacteria	Parasites
rotavirus: common in infants and young children	salmonella	giardia
norovirus: common in older children and adults	campylobacter	cryptosporidium
adenovirus	*Escherichia coli* (E. coli).	

Recognising the symptoms

The two hallmark symptoms of gastroenteritis are:

- diarrhoea (watery or loose stools)
- vomiting.

Other common symptoms

- **Nausea and stomach cramps:** These can range from mild discomfort to more intense pain.
- **Fever:** A low-grade fever is common, but high fevers can also occur.
- **Fatigue and weakness:** Your child might be less active and sleepier than usual.
- **Loss of appetite:** It's normal for children with gastroenteritis to not feel like eating.

The typical course of gastroenteritis

The duration of gastroenteritis can vary depending on the cause, but most viral infections last a few days to a week. Symptoms typically start one to three days after exposure and gradually improve over time.

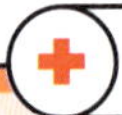

SEEK MEDICAL HELP

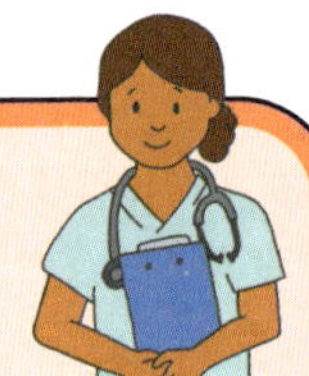

Consult your doctor if your child:

- has bloody diarrhoea or vomit
- shows signs of dehydration (dry mouth, sunken eyes, no tears when crying, decreased urination)
- has such perfuse, persistent watery diarrhoea that you are concerned about their hydration, even in the absence of signs of dehydration
- has a high fever (above 38.5°C) that persists for more than a few days
- has severe abdominal pain
- is unable to keep down any fluids
- has a weakened immune system or underlying medical conditions.

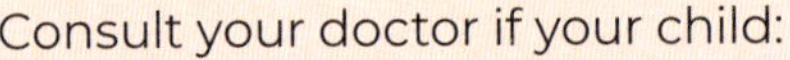

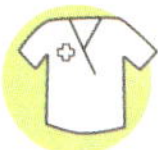

Treatment and management at home

The primary goal of treatment is to prevent dehydration, which can be a serious complication, especially in young children.

Here's what you can do:

- **Hydration:** Offer your child frequent sips of clear fluids like water, oral rehydration solutions, clear broth or diluted juice. Avoid sugary drinks, as they can worsen diarrhoea.
- **Bland diet:** Once vomiting subsides, gradually introduce bland foods like toast, rice or bananas. Avoid sugary, fatty, spicy foods and dairy.
- **Rest:** Make sure your child gets plenty of rest, as their body needs energy to fight off the infection.
- **Fever reducers:** If your child has a fever, you can give them paracetamol or ibuprofen as directed by your doctor or pharmacist.

Recovery

Another important thing to remember is that your child may struggle to process lactose for two to three weeks after a bout of gastro. This is called post-infectious lactose intolerance, where the original gastro resolves but nausea and diarrhoea persist for weeks afterwards. So go easy on the dairy, or consider a lactase substitute – you can discuss this with your local doctor.

Prevention

To reduce the risk of your child getting or spreading gastroenteritis, ensure:

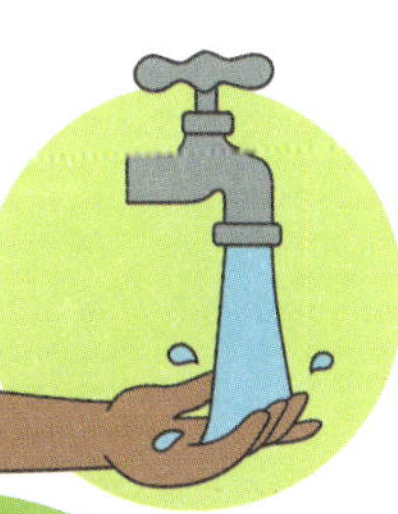

- **Hand hygiene:** Encourage frequent handwashing with soap and water, especially before eating and after using the toilet.
- **Food safety:** Cook food thoroughly, wash fruits and vegetables, and avoid raw or undercooked meat and eggs.
- **Clean surfaces:** Disinfect frequently touched surfaces regularly.

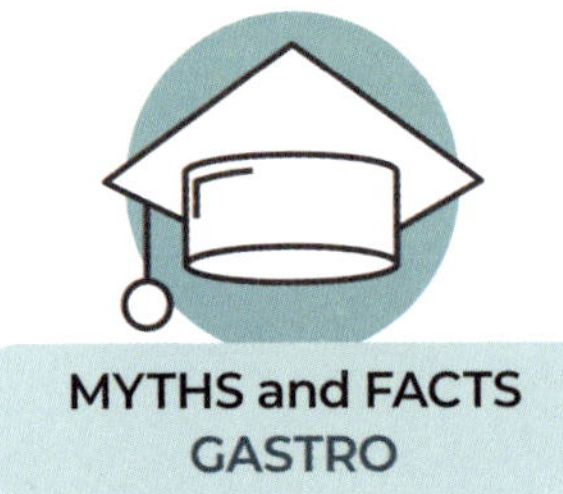

Myth: All stomach bugs are the same.

Fact: Gastroenteritis can be caused by different viruses, bacteria or parasites, each with slightly different symptoms, timelines and treatments.

Myth: You need to starve a child with gastroenteritis.

Fact: While it's important to avoid heavy or greasy foods, your child still needs fluids and nutrition.

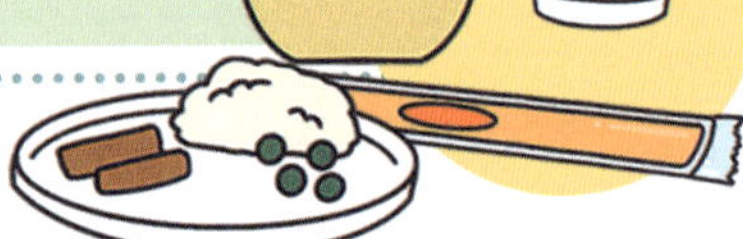

Childcare or school exclusion

Most childcare centres and schools devise their own policy regarding when kids can return. The safest rule of thumb is to delay return until forty-eight hours after the last loose bowel action or vomit.

Remember: Most children with gastroenteritis recover fully with at-home care. However, if you're ever concerned about your child's health or you have any questions, don't hesitate to reach out to your paediatrician. We're here to support you and your child's wellbeing.

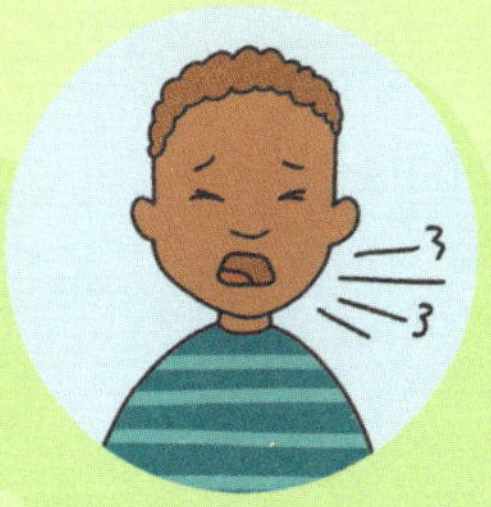

Upper respiratory illnesses

Upper respiratory illnesses

The common cold

Fellow parents! If you've ever felt like your child's nose is a never-ending fountain of snot, you're not alone. Colds and runny noses are an inevitability for most children, especially during the cooler months.

SYMPTOMS: THROAT TICKLE, RUNNY NOSE, SNEEZING, COUGH, SORE THROAT, LOW-GRADE FEVER, FATIGUE, IRRITABILITY, WATERY EYES, HEADACHES

What is the common cold?

The common cold isn't a single illness but a collection of viral infections that affect the upper respiratory tract, which includes the nose, throat, ears and sinuses. While more than 200 different viruses can cause the common cold, rhinoviruses are the most frequent culprits. These viruses are highly contagious and spread easily through the air when an infected person coughs or sneezes, or through direct contact with contaminated surfaces.

Who is most at risk of the common cold?

Children are particularly prone to catching colds due to their developing immune systems and close contact with other children in settings like childcare and school. On average, young children can experience up to twelve colds per year and older children six to eight per year, while adults typically have two to three.

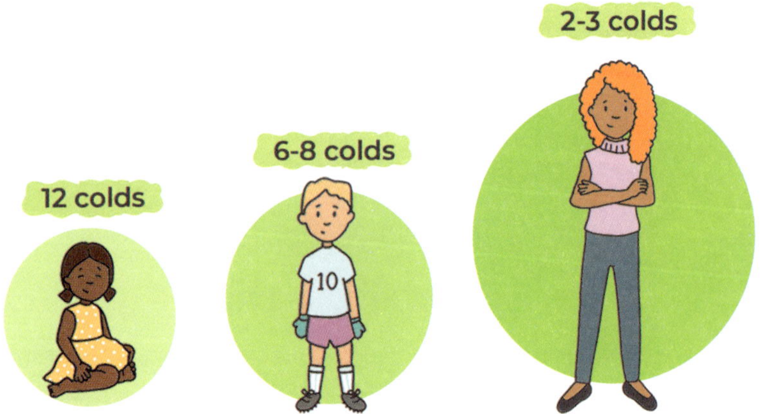

Why are children so prone to colds?
Young children are more susceptible to colds for a few reasons:

1. **Developing immune systems:** Their immune systems are still learning how to fight off viruses, so they catch colds more easily than adults.
2. **Close contact:** Kids are often in close contact with other children at childcare or school, making it easy for germs to spread.
3. **Developmental stage:** Young children are more likely to play on the floor, crawl on their hands, and bring objects, toys or food straight to their mouths. Given that bugs live on the floor, it should come as no surprise that children of this age get frequent infections.
4. **Hygiene habits:** Let's face it, little ones aren't always the best at handwashing or covering their mouths when they cough or sneeze!

Recognising the symptoms

The common cold often starts with a tickle in the throat or a runny/stuffy nose, which can progress to:

- sneezing
- cough
- sore throat
- low-grade fever
- fatigue
- irritability
- watery eyes
- headaches.

These symptoms usually peak within two to three days and gradually resolve over seven to ten days. Some children may only experience a snotty nose. And while a snotty nose might be the most visible symptom, it's actually a good thing! Mucus helps trap and remove germs from the body.

Once the cold has passed, it's common for a cough to linger (even for a happy, recovered child) for up to three weeks – this is when it can feel like you're on the merry-go-round of lurgies. A post-infectious cough and in an otherwise well child is harmless. Remember – this stage doesn't last forever.

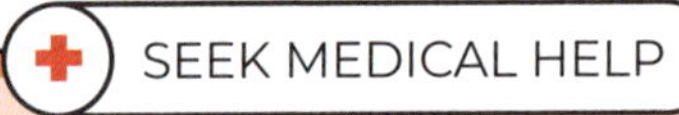

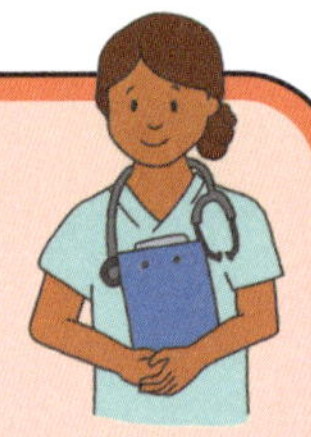

Most colds are mild and resolve on their own. However, you should consult your doctor if your child:

- is under three months old and has a fever
- has a high fever (above 38.5°C) which lasts for more than a few days
- has difficulty breathing, is wheezing or has a persistent cough
- shows signs of dehydration (dry mouth, fewer wet nappies, no tears when crying)
- doesn't improve after ten to fourteen days, or symptoms worsen
- has ear pain
- seems unusually lethargic or irritable.

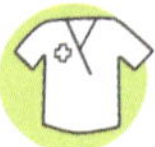

Treatment and management at home

There's no cure for the common cold, but there are plenty of things you can do to help your child feel better and manage their symptoms:

- **Hydration:** Encourage your child to drink plenty of fluids, such as water, breastmilk, formula, oral rehydration solution or clear broth. This helps keep them hydrated and can loosen mucus.
- **Saline:** Saline drops or spray can help loosen mucus and soothe irritated nasal passages. Then use a nasal aspirator for young children.
- **Humidifier:** A cool-mist humidifier can moisten the air and make breathing easier.

- **Pain and fever relief:** If your child has a fever or is uncomfortable, over-the-counter medications like paracetamol or ibuprofen can be helpful. Always follow the recommended dosage for your child's age and weight.
- **Rest:** Make sure your child gets plenty of rest, as their body needs energy to fight off the virus.
- **Elevate the head of the bed:** Slightly elevating the head of your child's bed can help with drainage and make breathing easier at night. This is not advised for babies. Always ensure you are following safe-sleep tips for younger children.

Prevention

While it's difficult to completely avoid the common cold, you can reduce the risk of your child getting sick by:

1. **Teaching good hand hygiene:** Encourage frequent handwashing with soap and water, especially after blowing noses, coughing or sneezing.
2. **Avoiding close contact with sick individuals:** Keep your child away from people who are sick.
3. **Cleaning and disinfecting surfaces:** Regularly clean and disinfect frequently touched surfaces, such as toys, doorknobs and countertops.

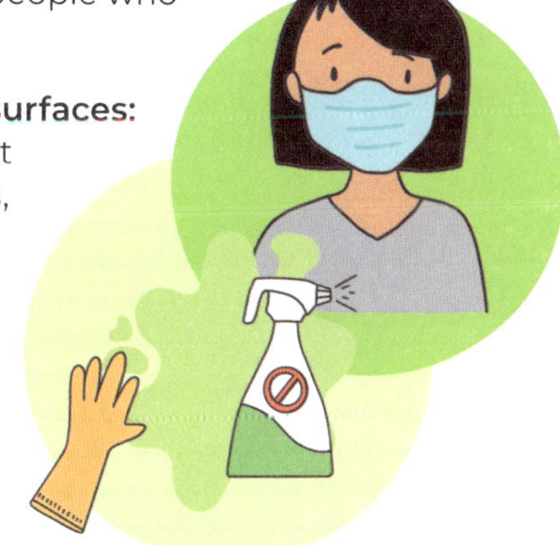

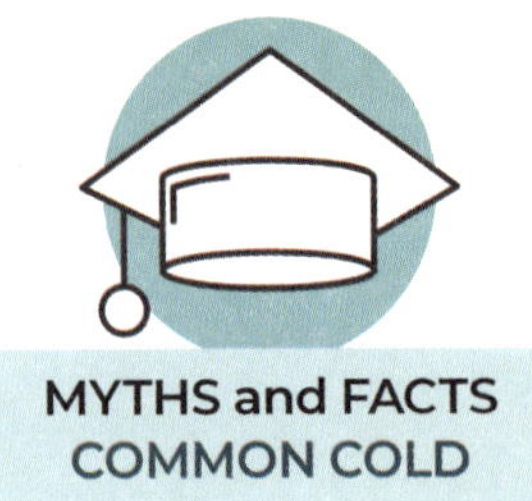

Myth: Antibiotics cure the common cold.

Fact: Antibiotics only work against bacteria, not viruses. Colds are caused by viruses, so antibiotics won't help.

Myth: Going out in cold weather causes colds.

Fact: You catch a cold by being exposed to the cold virus, not by being cold. However, cold weather can dry out the nasal passages, making it easier for viruses to take hold. Colder, wetter weather also encourages more 'inside play', where children are likely to be in closer proximity, making it easier for bugs to spread, which is why they cluster more in the winter months. Viruses also theoretically live longer on surfaces during colder weather, so it's worth wiping down toys and cleaning other surfaces when someone is unwell, to reduce further transmission.

Childcare or school exclusion

It's difficult to give advice on this, as each education setting will have developed their own policies and guidelines. As a general rule, if your child needs fever- or pain-reducing medication to feel 'well enough' to attend childcare or school, they should **not** be sent. Always be considerate towards the other children, their families, and the staff and educators.

Upper respiratory illnesses

Congestion

SYMPTOMS: RUNNY NOSE, NOISY OR FAST BREATHING, SNORING, SNEEZING, COUGHING

First-aid kit:

- nasal aspirator (snot sucker)
- saline spray or drops

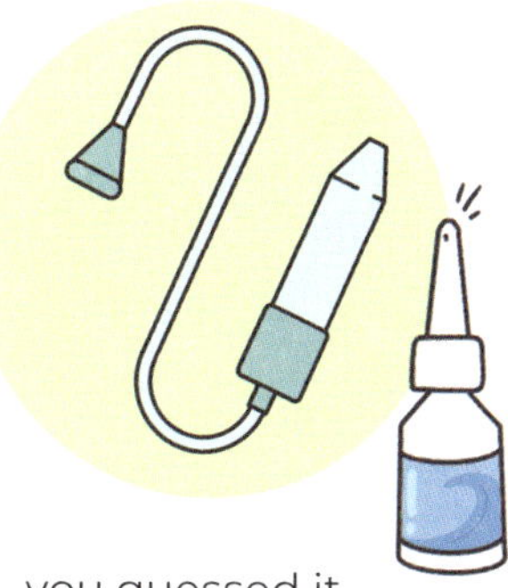

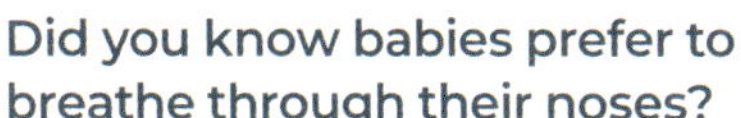

Did you know babies prefer to breathe through their noses?

Newborns are obligate nose breathers, meaning they primarily breathe through ... you guessed it, their noses!

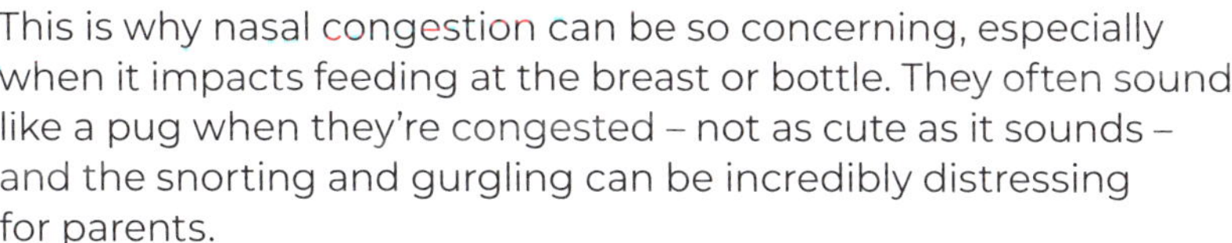

This is why nasal congestion can be so concerning, especially when it impacts feeding at the breast or bottle. They often sound like a pug when they're congested – not as cute as it sounds – and the snorting and gurgling can be incredibly distressing for parents.

Because children's nasal passages are small and therefore prone to congestion, three problems quickly emerge:

1. Breathing can be impaired.
2. Feeding can be impeded.
3. Sleep disturbances and general fussiness may result.

So there's good reason to be concerned about your baby's stuffy nose.

What causes newborn congestion?

These are the top three causes of excessive newborn congestion:

1. **Colds and respiratory infections (by far the most common cause):** Newborns have developing immune systems, making them susceptible to colds and respiratory infections. This can lead to an increase in mucus production and congestion, making it harder for your baby to breathe nasally.
2. **Environmental factors:** Dust, pet dander and other allergens in the air can irritate your baby's nose, leading to congestion.
3. **Dry air:** Dry air can irritate your baby's nose, leading to congestion. This is especially common during the winter months when heaters are in use.

Recognising the symptoms

- runny nose
- sniffling
- noisy or fast breathing
- snoring
- sneezing (this is your baby's natural way of clearing the mucus)
- coughing

Poor feeding can also lead to dehydration, fussiness and poor sleep.

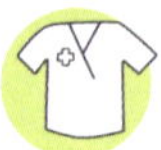

Treatment and management at home

The typical course of nasal congestion

Congestion often resolves within ten to fourteen days.

If your baby's congestion persists for more than two weeks or is accompanied by other concerning symptoms, such as a high fever, significant chestiness or difficulty breathing, seek medical advice.

A cough will often last longer than a runny nose if your baby has both symptoms. Remember, it's best to always consult your baby's healthcare provider if your little one has a cough or fever, especially if younger than three months old.

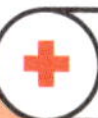

SEEK URGENT MEDICAL HELP

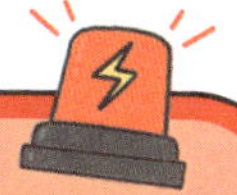

You should seek urgent medical assistance and present to ED or urgent care for:

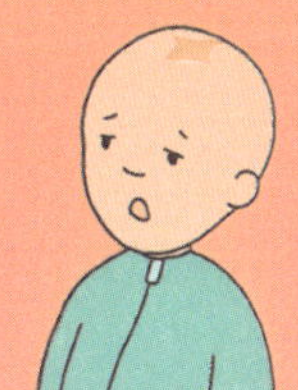

1. **Dehydration:** A baby who is fussy and isn't feeding can quickly become dehydrated. Signs your baby is dehydrated are dry nappies, no tears when crying, dry mouth, sunken eyes, a sunken fontanelle and general lethargy.

2. **Breathing difficulties:** Your baby might be having significant trouble breathing if they show signs of increased work of breathing, including flaring nostrils, grunting, or their chest and neck seem to be retracting with each breath.

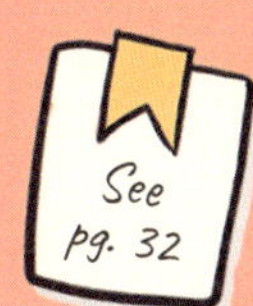

3. **Breathing faster than normal:** Babies already breathe quite fast – forty breaths per minute. If your baby is taking more than sixty breaths per minute or appears to have trouble catching their breath, you should call an ambulance.

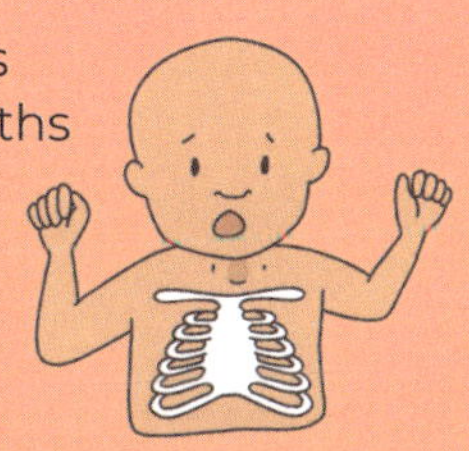

4. **Change in skin colour:** If you notice any change in your baby's skin colour, like a bluish tint around the lips, fingers or toes, this can indicate a lack of oxygen.

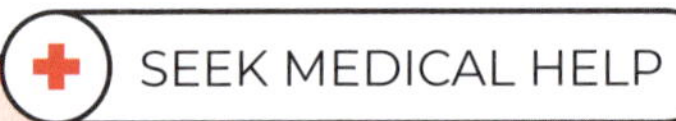

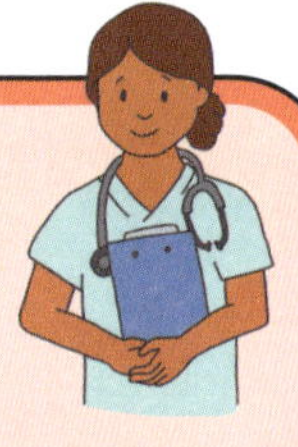

While newborn congestion is common and usually resolves on its own, there are instances where medical help may be necessary. You should consult your doctor if you notice:

1. **Persistent symptoms:** If the congestion persists for more than ten to fourteen days without any sign of improvement. This could indicate an underlying issue that needs medical attention.
2. **Fever:** If your baby develops a fever, especially if they are less than three months old. A fever in a newborn can be a sign of a more serious infection.
3. **Difficulty in feeding or sleeping:** If congestion is causing your baby significant difficulty in feeding, leading to poor weight gain, or trouble sleeping.
4. **High-pitched sounds:** Normal nasal congestion is associated with lower gurgles; high-pitched or squeaky sounds can be caused by a condition called laryngomalacia (discuss this with your baby's doctor). They could also be a sign of croup. I recommend all high-pitched sounds be reviewed.
5. **Unusual crying or irritability:** If your baby is unusually fussy or crying more than usual, or seems to be experiencing discomfort, this could be a sign that the congestion is causing significant distress.
6. **Chest congestion:** If you can hear or feel chest congestion, always have this reviewed.
7. **Other symptoms:** If congestion is accompanied by other symptoms, like a severe cough, vomiting or diarrhoea.
8. **Parental instinct:** If there's anything that seems off about your baby that is making you concerned – a parent's instinct is seldom wrong.

Congestion first aid

Step 1: Use saline nose drops.

- Saline drops can help loosen the mucus in your baby's nose, making it easier to clear.
- You can use specialised drops or a small syringe with saline solution.
- For older children you can use saline sprays.
- Lay your baby on their back and gently squeeze a few drops of saline solution into each nostril.
- Wait for a few moments.

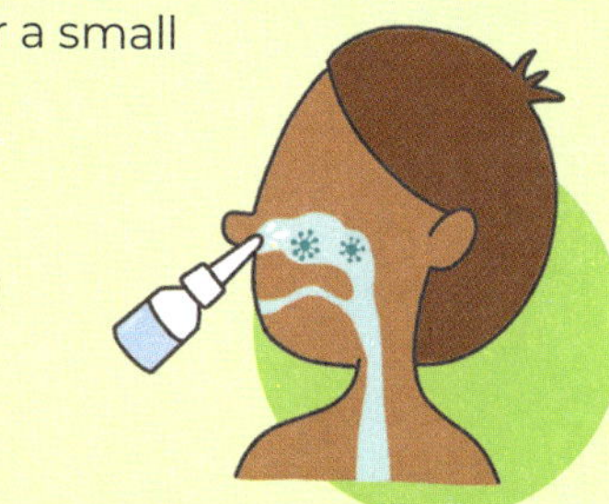

Step 2: Use a nasal aspirator (also known as a snot sucker) to suction out the loosened mucus.

- These devices help by removing excess mucus from your baby's nasal passages.

NOTE: Snot sucking will be one of the most disgustingly enjoyable things you'll do as a parent!

Option 1:

Manual snot suckers, where you use your own mouth on a hose to literally 'suck the snot' out of the nose. If you're like me, you'll prefer this option for better control, but the electric ones are great too. A filter protects you from any surprises entering your own mouth.

Option 2:

Electric snot suckers, for those who find the manual ones too difficult to use, or downright icky.

Option 3:

Bulb syringes. Squeeze the bulb, gently insert the tip into your baby's nostril, create a good seal, and release the bulb to deliver suction. Be careful not to insert the syringe too far into your baby's nose, but ensure there is a good seal within the nostril.

As a paediatrician, I can't recommend specific pharmaceuticals or medical devices, but every family with a baby needs saline and a snot-sucking aspirator of some description in their baby first-aid kit.

How often should I use saline and an aspirator?

If your baby is showing signs of congestion I recommend you use saline and an aspirator:

1. before every feed
2. before you put them down to sleep.

Other remedies to relieve newborn congestion

- **Steamy bathroom:** Create a steamy environment in your bathroom by running a hot shower. Sit in the bathroom with your baby for a few minutes to help loosen the mucus in their nose.
- **Humidifier:** Using a humidifier in your baby's room can add moisture to the air and help relieve congestion. Ensure that the humidifier is placed at a safe distance from your baby's cot to prevent any accidents. Don't add essential oils.
- **Give your baby a gentle face massage:** Very gently massage your baby's face – down their eyebrows, cheekbones, nose and temples. This can help warm and release mucus – plus your physical touch is highly comforting.

It's important to note that natural remedies may not work for every baby and consulting with your doctor or paediatrician is always recommended.

Monitoring hydration is key

Ensuring your baby stays well hydrated is important, especially if they are feeding less due to the congestion. Monitor their feeds – small amounts more often. Breastfeeding provides hydration, comfort and immune benefits that can help fight off infections. You can also use an oral rehydration solution in a small syringe in between feeds.

Newborn nasal congestion: what not to do

Don't stick a cotton bud up your baby's nose to try to clear the mucus out. If there is snot up there, allow it to be gently removed with saline and an aspirator. If your baby has had a viral swab you'll know it can cause bleeding and discomfort, so avoid cotton buds if possible.

Do not use medication, essential oils or vapour rubs. Most over-the-counter cold medications are not safe or effective for babies. Vapour rubs (often containing menthol, eucalyptus or camphor) are proven to be dangerous for children younger than two, and essential oils can be dangerous around young children.

With the right care and attention, you can help your congested newborn feed well, sleep better and thrive as they recover from whatever lurgy they have caught along the way.

Remember: It's always better to err on the side of caution when it comes to your baby's health, particularly with newborns. If you're concerned about your baby's nasal congestion, get your child's healthcare provider to take a look.

RSV: respiratory syncytial virus

RSV is regularly the culprit behind the common cold in children and seldom causes significant illness, but it can be particularly dangerous for very young babies. Thousands of babies with RSV are admitted to hospitals each year for breathing problems and asthma exacerbations, and premature, young babies are at the highest risk.

SYMPTOMS: WHEEZING, RAPID BREATHING, DIFFICULTY BREATHING, PERSISTENT COUGH, DECREASED APPETITE, LETHARGY

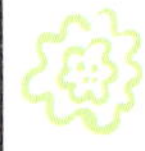

What is RSV?

RSV is a very common virus that affects the respiratory system, primarily the lungs and breathing passages. It's so common that most children will have had an RSV infection by the time they turn two. In older children and adults, RSV usually causes mild cold-like symptoms, but in infants and young children, it can lead to more serious illnesses like bronchiolitis, an inflammation of the small airways in the lungs.

Who is most at risk of RSV?

Infants and young children are particularly vulnerable to RSV, especially those born prematurely, with underlying heart or lung conditions, or with weakened immune systems. RSV is most prevalent during the cooler months, from late autumn to early spring.

Recognising the symptoms

The initial symptoms of RSV often resemble a common cold, including a runny nose, cough and sometimes low-grade fever. However, as the infection progresses, you may notice:

- **Wheezing:** A high-pitched whistling sound when your child breathes.
- **Rapid breathing:** Breathing faster than usual.
- **Difficulty breathing:** This can manifest as your child's chest pulling in with each breath (retractions), flaring of their nostrils or grunting sounds.
- **Persistent cough:** The cough might produce mucus or phlegm. It is really distinctive – like a chain-smoker's raspy cough. I often hear it from my waiting room and you can diagnose it from a distance!
- **Decreased appetite:** Your child may have difficulty feeding or drinking.
- **Lethargy:** They might seem unusually tired or less active.

The typical course of RSV

RSV infections usually follow a predictable pattern. The first few days your child might present with mild cold-like symptoms, which can then worsen into coughing, wheezing and difficulty breathing. The illness typically peaks around days five to seven, after which symptoms improve over the following week or two.

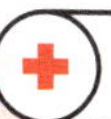

SEEK MEDICAL HELP

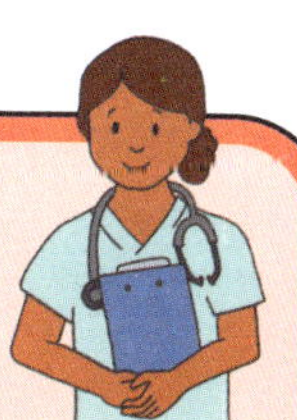

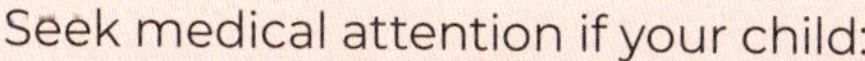

Seek medical attention if your child:

- has difficulty breathing or is breathing very rapidly
- has blue lips or fingernails
- is unusually drowsy or difficult to wake up
- refuses to feed or drink, or shows signs of dehydration (dry mouth, fewer wet nappies, no tears when crying)
- has an underlying health condition that puts them at higher risk of complications.

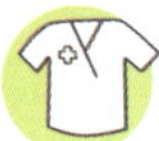

Treatment and management at home

There are ways to support your child's recovery at home:

- **Hydration:** Ensure your child is well hydrated by offering plenty of fluids, such as breastmilk, formula or water (for older children).
- **Clear airways:** A cool-mist humidifier can help moisten the air and loosen mucus. Saline nose drops (and snot suckers for babies and younger children) can also help clear nasal passages.

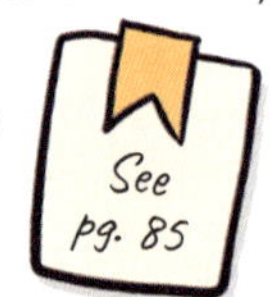

- **Comfort measures:** If your child has a fever, you can give them paracetamol or ibuprofen as recommended by your doctor or pharmacist. Ensure they get plenty of rest.

Prevention

The fantastic news is that immunisation against RSV is offered to pregnant women (antibodies against RSV can easily pass through the placenta) and many countries, including Australia, now offer RSV monoclonal antibodies to eligible infants after birth. This monoclonal antibody has been shown to reduce hospitalisations by 90 per cent.

At home, there are steps you can take to reduce the risk of RSV infection:

- **Hand hygiene:** Wash your hands often, especially before touching your child.
- **Avoid close contact with sick individuals:** Limit your child's exposure to people with cold- or flu-like symptoms.
- **Clean surfaces:** Disinfect frequently touched surfaces regularly.

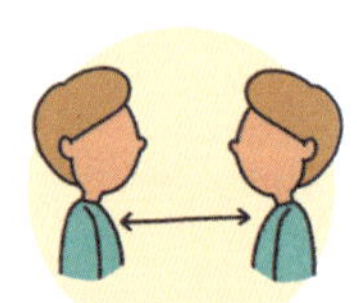

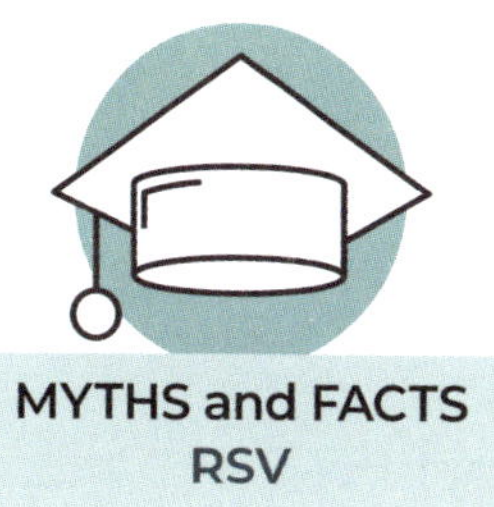

MYTHS and FACTS RSV

Myth: Antibiotics can cure RSV.

Fact: RSV is a viral infection, not a bacterial one, so antibiotics are not effective.

Myth: All wheezing in children means asthma.

Fact: While wheezing is a common symptom of asthma, it can also be caused by RSV and other respiratory conditions. A diagnosis of asthma is seldom given under two years of age.

Childcare or school exclusion

It is best to keep your child home until they are well again.

Remember: Most children with RSV recover fully at home with supportive care. However, if you're ever worried about your child's condition, trust your instincts and seek medical advice. We're here to help!

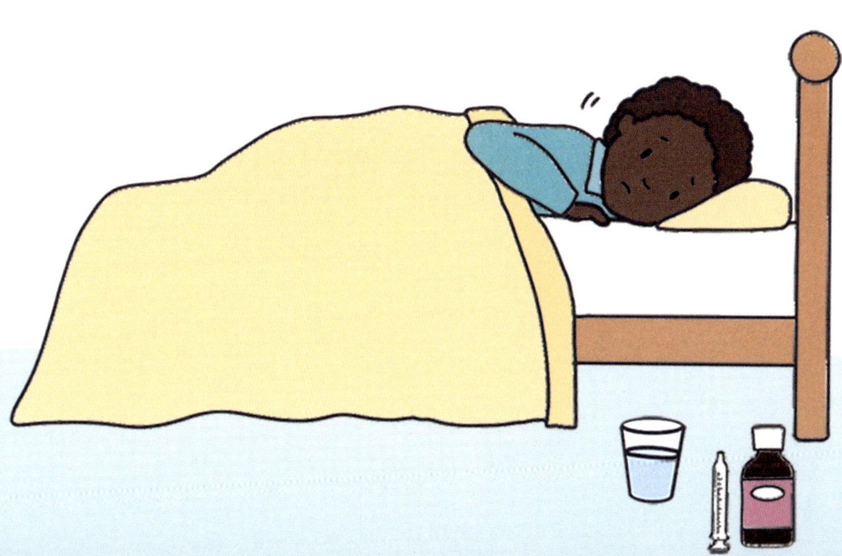

Bronchiolitis

Bronchiolitis is a common respiratory condition that affects infants and young children, especially during the winter months. While it can be a worrying time for parents and caregivers, understanding this condition and knowing how to manage it can make a world of difference for your little one. I find the best way to describe bronchiolitis is: *the common cold for a baby in the first year of life*. The two major concerns to focus on are hydration and work of breathing.

SYMPTOMS: WHEEZING, RAPID BREATHING, DIFFICULTY BREATHING, PERSISTENT COUGH, CHANGES IN EATING AND DRINKING, LETHARGY

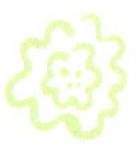

What is bronchiolitis?

Bronchiolitis is an inflammation of the tiny airways in the lungs called bronchioles. Bronchiolitis is not an infection itself, but rather a response to an infection – there are many potential bugs that can trigger an episode.

Think of the lungs as being like an upside-down tree. The main trunk is the trachea – or windpipe – which divides into two to deliver oxygen to both lungs, then divides again, multiple times, so it looks like small branches and twigs. We call these airways bronchioles.

Bronchiolitis is most often caused by a virus, usually the respiratory syncytial virus (RSV; see page 88), and inflammation leads to swelling and mucus build-up in those tiny airways, making it harder for young children to breathe effectively.

Who is most at risk of bronchiolitis?
Bronchiolitis primarily affects babies and young children, especially those younger than one year old. It's most common during the cooler months, from late autumn to early spring, and the offending bug can spread easily through close contact with someone who is sick.

 Recognising the symptoms

In its early stages, bronchiolitis often looks like a common cold: a runny nose, cough and sometimes a low-grade fever. Most cases last seven to ten days – with the worst symptoms on day three – and resolve rapidly without complication.

If the infection progresses, though, your child might develop:

- **Wheezing:** A high-pitched whistling sound when they breathe.
- **Rapid breathing:** You'll notice their little chest moving up and down much faster than usual.
- **Difficulty breathing:** Look for signs like their nostrils flaring out, their tummy sucking in under their ribs, or grunting sounds with each breath.
- **A persistent cough:** This cough might bring up mucus.
- **Changes in eating and drinking:** They may have less appetite and struggle to feed or drink normally.
- **Lethargy:** They might seem more tired or less active than usual.

The typical course of bronchiolitis
Bronchiolitis generally follows a pattern:

- **Days one and two:** Cold-like symptoms such as a runny nose and cough.
- **Days three to five:** The coughing and wheezing gets worse, and breathing may become more difficult.
- **Days five to seven:** This is usually the peak of the illness, when symptoms are most severe.
- **The following week:** Symptoms gradually start to improve.

Most children recover fully within two weeks, although a cough can sometimes linger a bit longer.

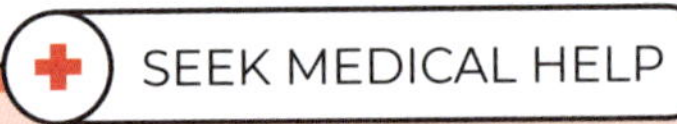

It's important to see a doctor if your child:

- has trouble breathing or is breathing very rapidly
- has blue lips or fingernails (a sign of not getting enough oxygen)
- seems very drowsy or difficult to wake up
- refuses to feed or drink, or is showing signs of dehydration like fewer wet nappies or a dry mouth
- or if you are concerned at any point.

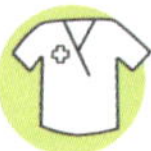

Treatment and management at home

There's no specific cure for bronchiolitis, but there are plenty of things you can do at home to help your child feel more comfortable:

1. **Hydration is key:** Offer your child plenty of fluids, like breastmilk or formula for babies, or water for older children.
2. **Clear airways:** Use a cool-mist humidifier to moisten the air and help loosen mucus. Saline drops can also help clear their nose.
3. **Comfort measures:** If they have a fever, give them paracetamol or ibuprofen as directed by your doctor or pharmacist. Make sure they get plenty of rest.

Prevention

Steps to take to reduce the risk of your child getting or spreading the bugs that can cause bronchiolitis:

1. **Handwashing:** Wash your hands often and encourage everyone in the family to do the same.
2. **Avoid sick contacts:** Try to limit your child's exposure to people who are unwell.

3. **Clean surfaces:** Regularly clean and disinfect surfaces that are touched frequently, like toys and doorknobs.

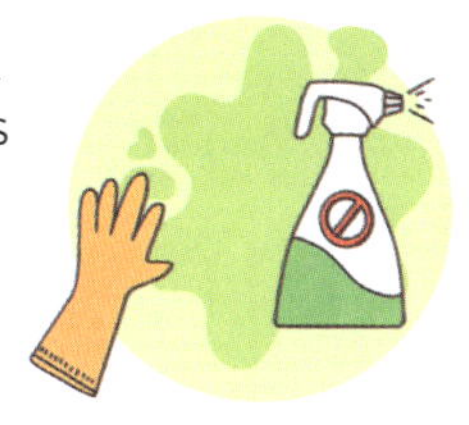

4. **Vaccinations:** Ensure your child is up to date with their routine vaccinations, including the flu shot and RSV immunisation (for pregnant women and children).

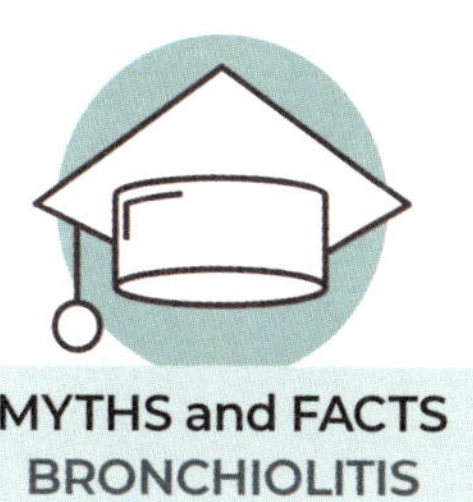

MYTHS and FACTS
BRONCHIOLITIS

Myth: All wheezing in children means asthma.

Fact: While wheezing is a common symptom of asthma, it can also be caused by bronchiolitis and other respiratory conditions.

Myth: Antibiotics can cure bronchiolitis.

Fact: Bronchiolitis is usually caused by a virus, not bacteria, so antibiotics seldom help.

Childcare or school exclusion

It is best to keep them home until they are well again. The cough may linger in an otherwise well child, but they can return to childcare or school if they are eating and drinking well and not requiring pain or fever-reducing medication.

Remember: Most children with bronchiolitis recover fully with at-home care, but always trust your instincts as a parent. If you're worried about your child, don't hesitate to seek medical advice. We're here to help you and your child through this.

Upper respiratory illnesses

Influenza

As a paediatrician, one of the most common illnesses I see during the colder months is influenza, colloquially known as the flu. While it often behaves like the common cold, influenza can escalate to a quite nasty infection in some adults and children, and can be especially dangerous in young babies, the elderly and those with underlying health conditions. The flu can also weaken the immune system and leave children vulnerable to opportunistic bacterial infections.

SYMPTOMS: HIGH FEVER, CHILLS, BODY ACHES, HEADACHE, FATIGUE, COUGH, SORE THROAT, RUNNY NOSE, VOMITING, DIARRHOEA

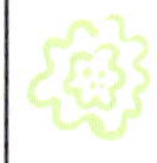

What is influenza?

The flu is not just a common cold; it is caused by the influenza virus, and it's not to be taken lightly. It's a respiratory illness that can cause a whole host of unpleasant symptoms, like the common cold but to the extreme.

- **High fever:** This often comes on suddenly and can last several days.
- **Chills:** Your little one might feel shivery, even under warm blankets.
- **Body aches:** Muscles can feel sore and ache all over.
- **Headache:** Often described as pounding or throbbing.
- **Fatigue:** The flu can really wipe kids out, leaving them feeling exhausted.
- **Cough, sore throat, runny nose:** These classic cold symptoms are usually present too.
- **Vomiting and diarrhoea:** These are more common in younger children.

How does the influenza spread?

The flu virus is a social butterfly, spreading easily through:

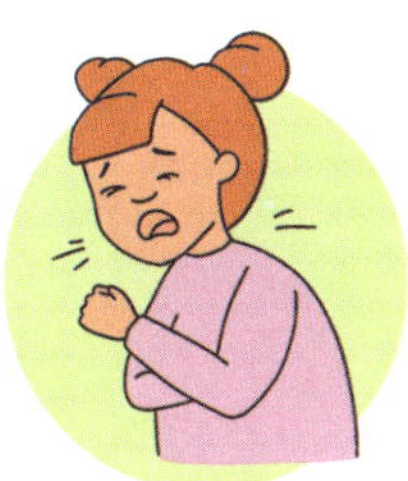

- **Droplets:** When someone with the flu coughs or sneezes, tiny droplets containing the virus go flying!
- **Direct contact:** If your child touches contaminated surfaces then touches their eyes, nose or mouth. Good hand hygiene is important!

The typical course of influenza

The flu typically lasts about a week, but some kids might take a little longer to recover fully. The first few days are usually the worst, with symptoms gradually improving. Don't be surprised if their energy levels take a few weeks to return to normal after the flu.

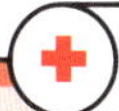

SEEK MEDICAL HELP

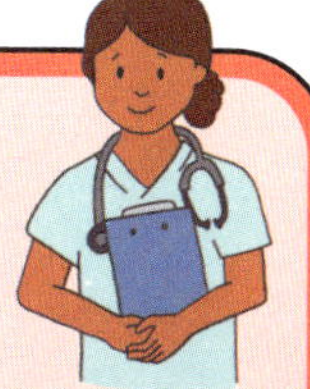

While most kids recover from the flu at home, here's when you should call your local doctor:

- Your child is under two years old.
- They have a chronic illness (like asthma or diabetes). An antiviral medication for influenza does exist, although it is only used in specific circumstances.
- They have difficulty breathing.
- Their fever gets very high or doesn't come down with medication.
- They seem very dehydrated (dry mouth, no tears, less urine).
- Their symptoms get worse after improving. Although uncommon, there is a chance your child might succumb to a bacterial infection while their body is 'distracted' fighting the flu. Any change for the worse should be reviewed by a doctor.

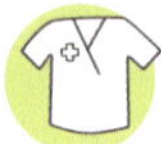

Treatment and management at home

There's no magic cure for the flu, but you can help your child feel more comfortable.

- **Rest:** Lots of it! Let them sleep as much as they need.
- **Fluids:** Offer water, clear broths, electrolyte drinks and icy poles to keep them hydrated.
- **Fever and pain relief:** Children's paracetamol or ibuprofen can help manage fever and aches.
- **Humidifier:** A cool-mist humidifier can soothe a sore throat and stuffy nose.

Prevention

The best way to protect your child is to get them vaccinated against the flu every year. This is possible from six months of age. Keep in mind that in the first year of getting vaccinated, they'll need two doses, one month apart. Good hand hygiene and avoiding close contact with sick people are also essential.

Childcare or school exclusion

It is best to keep them home until they are well again.

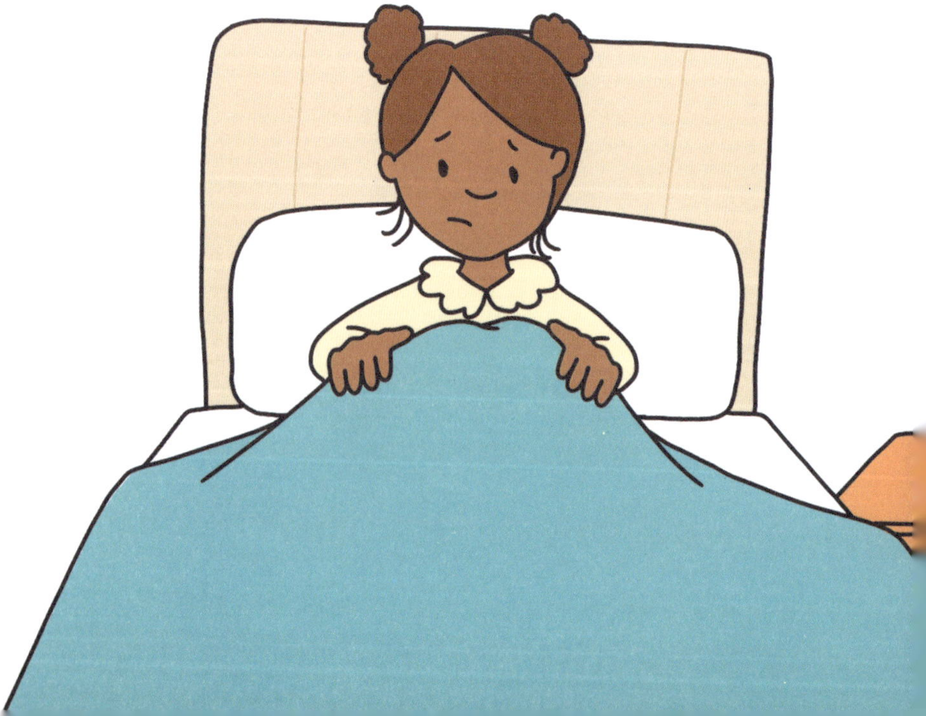

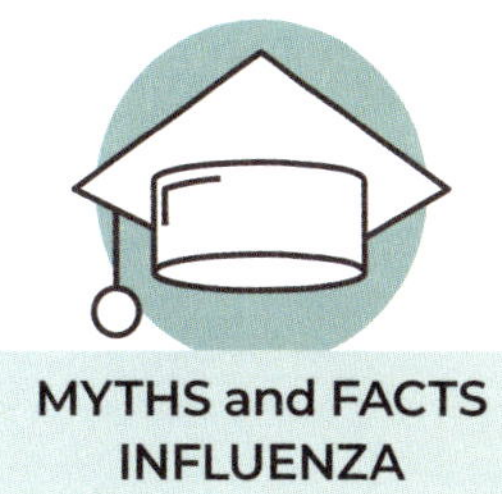

MYTHS and FACTS INFLUENZA

Myth: The flu is just a bad cold.

Fact: The flu is often much more intense, with higher fevers and more severe body aches. People who have experienced true influenza never refer to the common cold as the flu!

Myth: The flu shot gives you the flu.

Fact: The flu vaccine contains an inactivated virus that can't cause illness. It might cause some mild side effects, but nowhere near the actual symptoms of infection. It's the best way to protect against the flu.

Myth: Our family has had the flu vaccination, so there's no way we'll catch the flu this winter.

Fact: Certain vaccines are not 100 per cent protective, and influenza is one such vaccine. The annual vaccination only protects you against the variant that's been the most common around the world that season and it also wanes over time. It is still possible for a vaccinated child to catch the flu, but they'll likely have a shorter, less severe episode. Vaccination is still the best line of defence when it comes to the flu.

Remember: Don't hesitate to reach out to your local doctor if you have any concerns about your child's health. We're always here to help!

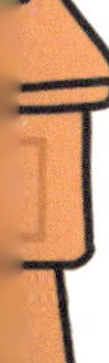

Croup

Croup is a common childhood illness known for its distinctive barking cough, which can sound very alarming. Similar to bronchiolitis, croup is a response to a bug, not an infection in itself. Rest assured, most cases are mild and can be managed effectively at home. Children can deteriorate incredibly rapidly, so it's crucial you keep an eye on them and, if you're concerned, seek medical review without delay. Let's explore what croup is, and how you can help your little one feel better.

SYMPTOMS: HOARSENESS, STRIDOR, DIFFICULTY BREATHING, FEVER, RUNNY NOSE, CONGESTION

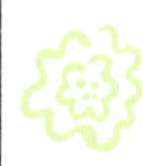

What is croup?

Croup is typically a response to a viral upper respiratory infection that causes swelling and inflammation in the larynx (voice box), trachea (windpipe) and bronchi (the airways leading to each lung). We call it laryngotracheobronchitis. This swelling leads to croup's characteristic cough, which can sound like a seal or a dog barking. Croup is most commonly caused by the parainfluenza virus, but other viruses can also be responsible.

Who is most at risk of croup?

Croup typically affects children between six months and three years old. It's more common during the winter months and the offending bugs spread easily through respiratory droplets when an infected person coughs or sneezes.

Recognising the symptoms

Scan here for stridor cough example

The hallmark symptom of croup is the barking cough, which is often worse at night. Some say this sounds similar to a barking seal. Other common symptoms include:

- **Hoarseness:** Your child's voice might sound raspy or weak.
- **Stridor:** A high-pitched whistling sound when your child breathes in, which is more noticeable when they are upset or crying.
- **Difficulty breathing:** While most cases of croup are mild, some children may experience difficulty breathing, especially at night.
- **Fever:** A low-grade fever is common, but not always present.
- **Runny nose and congestion:** These are often the first signs of croup, resembling a common cold.

The typical course of croup

Croup usually starts with cold-like symptoms and progresses to a barking cough, hoarseness and sometimes stridor. Symptoms typically worsen at night and can last for three to five days. Most children recover fully within a week.

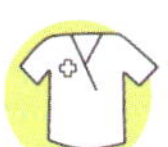

Treatment and management at home

Most cases of croup are mild and can be managed at home with support and care.

- **Comfort and reassurance:** Crying and agitation can worsen breathing difficulties so offer as much comfort to your child as they need so they're calm and settled.
- **Hydration:** Encourage your child to drink plenty of fluids to prevent dehydration.
- **Fever reducers:** If your child has a fever, you can give them paracetamol or ibuprofen as directed by your doctor or pharmacist.

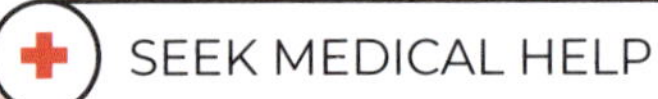

SEEK MEDICAL HELP

While most cases of croup are mild, it's important to seek medical attention if:

- your child is having difficulty breathing or their breathing is very fast or laboured
- you hear a high-pitched whistling sound when your child breathes in at rest (stridor)
- your child's lips or fingernails turn blue
- your child seems unusually drowsy or difficult to wake up
- your child's symptoms worsen or don't improve after a few days.

In some cases, your doctor may prescribe a dose of steroids to help reduce inflammation and ease breathing. Sometimes inhaled medicine is also used. A daily dose of steroid might be continued for three days in total and is entirely safe when used this way.

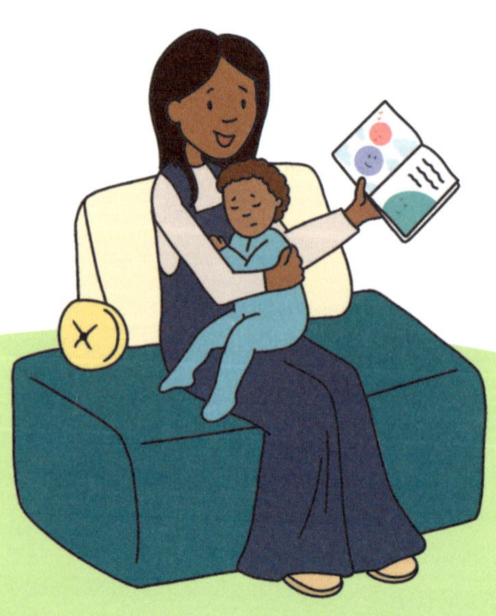

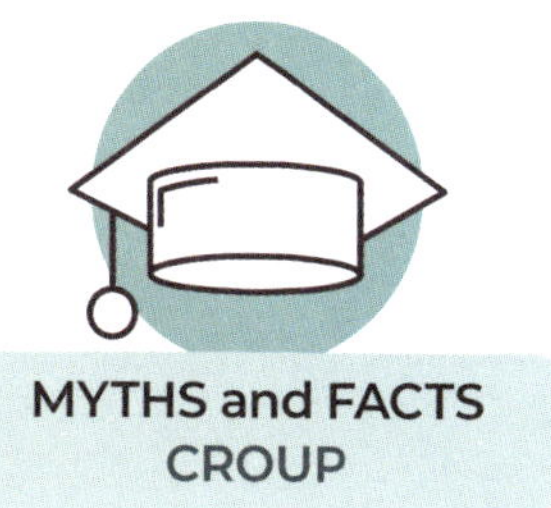

MYTHS and FACTS
CROUP

Myth: You can wait until morning to see the doctor.

Fact: Croup can worsen with very little warning. It is not advised to wait until morning if your child has croup and is showing any signs of deterioration or distress.

Myth: A warm shower will fix croup.

Fact: Recent scientific evidence shows that steam exposure is not useful as a croup treatment, but if your child enjoys the comfort of a warm shower or bath (especially together with a parent), then this is certainly advised. Just never leave a sick child (even older children) unattended near water.

Recurring croup

While a single episode of croup is common, some children have a tendency to get croup again and again. The treatment is similar and parents often request multiple prescriptions of steroid medicine 'just in case' – this is seldom advisable because each episode might be different and medical review is crucial.

Childcare or school exclusion

It is best to keep them home until they are well again.

Remember: Croup is a common childhood illness, and most children recover fully with at-home care. If you have any further questions or concerns, don't hesitate to reach out to your paediatrician. We're here to support you and your child on their health journey.

Strep throat

Arguably the most frequent symptom of childhood illness during the school year is a sore throat. While many sore throats are caused by mild viruses and resolve on their own, some are caused by a bacterial infection known colloquially as strep throat. It's important for parents to be aware of the signs, treatment and preventive measures for strep throat, to ensure their child gets the care they need.

SYMPTOMS: SUDDEN ONSET OF SORE THROAT, FEVER, PAINFUL SWALLOWING, RED AND SWOLLEN TONSILS, SWOLLEN LYMPH NODES

What is strep throat?

Strep throat, or streptococcal pharyngitis, is caused by a bacterium called group A streptococcus (group A strep). It's highly contagious and typically affects children between five and fifteen years old, though anyone can get it. Being a bacteria, it responds well to antibiotics.

How does strep throat spread?

Strep throat is primarily spread through direct contact with respiratory droplets from an infected person's cough or sneeze.

Recognising the symptoms

While a sore throat is the most common symptom of strep throat, it's crucial to distinguish it from a viral sore throat, which is often less severe and doesn't require antibiotics. Here's what to watch out for:

- **Sudden onset:** Strep throat often appears abruptly, while viral sore throats tend to develop more gradually.
- **Painful swallowing:** Your child may complain of pain or difficulty swallowing.

- **Fever:** A high fever (over 38°C) is frequently associated with strep throat.
- **Red and swollen tonsils:** The tonsils may appear red and swollen, and might have white patches or streaks of pus.
- **Swollen lymph nodes:** The lymph nodes in the neck might be enlarged and tender to the touch.
- **Other symptoms:** Your child may also experience headache, stomach pain, nausea, vomiting or a rash.

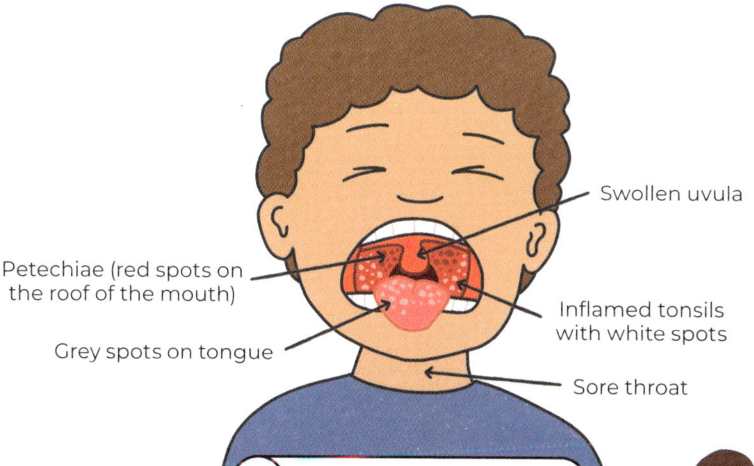

Swollen uvula

Petechiae (red spots on the roof of the mouth)

Inflamed tonsils with white spots

Grey spots on tongue

Sore throat

SEEK MEDICAL HELP

If your child shows any of these symptoms, and especially a combination of them, it's important to schedule an appointment with your local doctor. They can perform a rapid strep test or throat culture to confirm the diagnosis. The speed of this test is especially important, because antibiotics need to be started straight away.

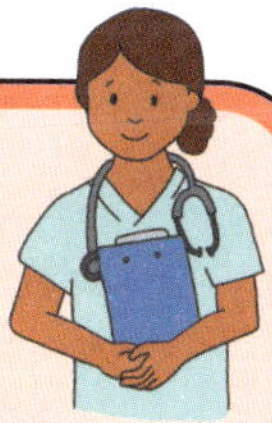

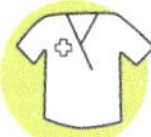

Treatment and management at home

Antibiotics are essential: unlike viral sore throats, strep throat requires treatment with antibiotics to prevent possible complications like rheumatic fever, kidney inflammation, and sinus or ear infections. Your child must complete the entire course of antibiotics as prescribed by their doctor, even if your child's symptoms improve before the recommended course finishes.

Easing the discomfort

While antibiotics work to fight the infection, you can help your child feel more comfortable with:

- **Pain relief:** Over-the-counter pain relievers like paracetamol or ibuprofen can alleviate pain and reduce fever.
- **Soothing fluids:** Warm liquids like broth, soup or herbal teas can help soothe a sore throat. Cold treats like icy poles or ice cream might also provide relief.
- **Humidifier:** A cool-mist humidifier can add moisture to the air, reducing throat irritation.

Protecting others: hygiene is key

- **Encourage good hand hygiene:** Teach your child to wash their hands often with soap and water for at least twenty seconds, especially after coughing or sneezing.
- **Cover coughs and sneezes:** Teach your child to use a tissue or their elbow to cover coughs and sneezes, and immediately dispose of used tissues.
- **Disinfect surfaces:** Regularly clean and disinfect frequently touched surfaces, such as toys, doorknobs and light switches.
- **Avoid sharing personal items:** Discourage your child from sharing drinks, utensils or personal items like toothbrushes.

A note about scarlet fever

In some cases, strep throat can lead to scarlet fever, a rash that appears as small red bumps and feels like sandpaper. This rash typically starts on the chest and stomach and spreads to other parts of the body. It's usually accompanied by a strawberry-like appearance of the tongue. If you notice these symptoms, contact your local doctor for diagnosis and treatment.

Childcare or school exclusion

Keep your child home until they have been on antibiotics for at least twenty-four hours and are fever-free.

Remember: Early detection and treatment are key to preventing complications from strep throat. If you have any concerns about your child's health, don't hesitate to reach out to your child's doctor. We're here to help!

Upper respiratory illnesses

Pneumonia

As a paediatrician, I often treat children with pneumonia, especially during the colder months. While it can be a serious illness, most kids recover quickly from uncomplicated pneumonia. Let's demystify pneumonia and discuss how to keep your little ones healthy.

SYMPTOMS: COUGH, FEVER, RAPID BREATHING, DIFFICULTY BREATHING, CHEST PAIN, FATIGUE, POOR APPETITE

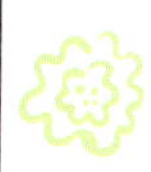

What is pneumonia?

Pneumonia is an infection of the lungs and, similar to bronchiolitis or croup, it is a response to a bug. The tiny air sacs in the lungs, called alveoli, become inflamed and filled with fluid, making it harder for the lungs to do their job, which is to get oxygen into – and carbon dioxide out of – the bloodstream. This can lead to a range of symptoms, from mild to severe.

Causes of pneumonia: it's not just one thing

Several culprits can cause pneumonia in children:

- **Viruses:** These are the most common cause, especially in younger children. Respiratory syncytial virus (RSV), influenza (flu) and rhinovirus (common cold) are frequent offenders.
- **Bacteria:** *Streptococcus pneumoniae* (pneumococcus) is the most common bacterial cause, and is vaccine preventable.
- **Other germs:** Less commonly, fungi or mycoplasma can cause atypical pneumonia.

How does pneumonia spread?

The common cold might cause a sniffle in one individual and full-blown pneumonia in another. Pneumonia-causing germs – like all respiratory bugs – are often spread through the air when an infected person coughs or sneezes. They can also spread through direct contact with respiratory secretions, like saliva or mucus.

Recognising the symptoms

While pneumonia can seem like a cold at first, it typically progresses to more severe symptoms, including:

- **Cough:** This can be dry or produce phlegm (mucus).
- **Fever:** Often high, but sometimes low-grade or even absent in young infants.
- **Rapid breathing:** You might notice your child's chest moving faster than usual or their nostrils flaring.
- **Difficulty breathing:** Your child may be working harder to breathe, grunting or wheezing.
- **Chest pain:** This can be worse with coughing or deep breaths.
- **Fatigue:** Your child may be unusually tired or less active.
- **Poor appetite:** Infants might have trouble feeding or complain of abdominal pain.

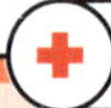

SEEK MEDICAL HELP

If your child has any of the following, it's important to seek medical attention promptly:

- difficulty breathing or fast breathing
- bluish lips or nails
- chest pain
- high fever that doesn't improve with medication
- dehydration (dry mouth, no tears, less urine)
- signs of severe illness (lethargy, confusion, irritability).

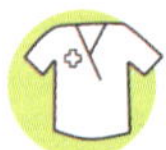

Treatment and management at home

Complications of pneumonia are treated independently; for example intravenous fluid might be used for severely dehydrated children. Treatment for pneumonia depends on the causative bug.

- **Viral pneumonia:** Most cases resolve on their own with rest and fluids. Your doctor may recommend fever-reducing medication to ease symptoms.
- **Bacterial pneumonia:** Antibiotics are the treatment of choice. Mild to moderate bacterial pneumonia can be managed at home with oral antibiotics, but sometimes intravenous antibiotics are needed.
- **Other causes:** Treatment will be tailored to the specific germ.

Prevention

While not all pneumonia can be prevented, here are some things you can do to reduce the risk:

1. **Vaccinations:** Ensure your child is up to date on their routine vaccinations, including pneumococcal and influenza vaccines.
2. **Hand hygiene:** Teach your child to wash their hands frequently and avoid touching their face, especially around meal times.
3. **Avoid sick contacts:** Keep your child away from people who are ill, especially during cold and flu season.
4. **Breastfeeding:** If possible, breastfeeding offers infants some protection against respiratory infections.

Childcare or school exclusion

There are no explicit guidelines about exclusion periods for pneumonia, due to the causes being so variable. If it's viral pneumonia, generally children can return to childcare or school once well again. If bacterial, then once they have been on twenty-four to forty-eight hours of appropriate antibiotics and are well enough in themselves, they should be okay to return to school. It is best to seek personal medical advice on return to childcare or school in this circumstance.

Remember: Pneumonia can be a serious illness, but with early diagnosis and appropriate treatment most children recover fully. You can't catch pneumonia, but you can catch the bug that might cause it, so stay up to date with vaccines, avoid sick contacts wherever possible and teach children to practise good hygiene – as much as is developmentally appropriate and possible for their age.

Whooping cough (pertussis)

The sound of a child's persistent cough can be incredibly distressing for parents. One cough pattern that can be particularly worrisome is the inspiratory 'whoop' of pertussis, also known as whooping cough. While pertussis is now much less common thanks to vaccinations, it's still important to be aware of it and to know how to protect your children – especially young babies.

SYMPTOMS: RUNNY NOSE, SNEEZING, COUGH

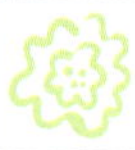

What is whooping cough?

Whooping cough is a highly contagious respiratory infection caused by the bacterium *Bordetella pertussis*. It's notorious for causing severe coughing spells that can be quite scary; in young infants, it's particularly dangerous because it can cause apnoeas – breathing pauses that can be fatal.

Whooping cough gets its name from the distinctive 'whoop' sound a child makes when breathing in rapidly, classically between runs of coughs (sometimes called coughing spasms, fits or paroxysms).

Why is whooping cough such a concern?

Before the development of a vaccine, whooping cough was a leading cause of infant deaths. While it's less common now, it can still pose a serious risk to babies and young children. Their airways are smaller and more easily blocked by mucus, making breathing difficult during coughing fits.

How does whooping cough spread?
Whooping cough spreads easily through respiratory droplets when an infected person coughs or sneezes. It's most contagious during the early stages of the illness, before the characteristic 'whoop' develops.

Who is most at risk of whooping cough?
Infants are at the highest risk of serious complications from whooping cough, especially those who haven't completed their full course of vaccinations.

Recognising the symptoms

- Whooping cough typically starts like a common cold, with a runny nose, sneezing and mild cough.
- After a week or two, the cough worsens and becomes more frequent, often occurring in intense bursts.
- These coughing fits can be followed by a high-pitched 'whoop' sound as the child gasps for air.
- Sometimes the coughing fits can be followed by a large vomit.
- The cough tends to ease in frequency and intensity after a few days, but may linger in a lesser form for several weeks. Colloquially, whooping cough was known as the 100-day cough, because it can literally hang around for more than three months!

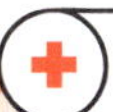

SEEK MEDICAL HELP

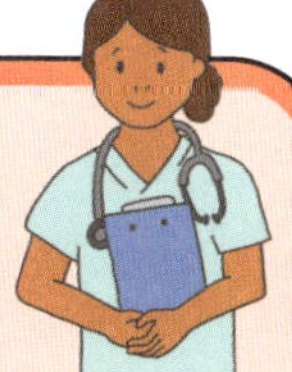

Don't hesitate to seek medical attention if your child:

- has a severe or persistent cough
- has difficulty breathing or turns blue during a coughing fit
- is vomiting or has difficulty feeding
- seems unusually sleepy or lethargic.

Prevention: how can I protect my child?

Vaccination is the most effective way to protect your child from whooping cough. The pertussis vaccine is usually given in combination with diphtheria and tetanus vaccines (DTaP) in a series of five doses during childhood. The greatest protection that can be provided to a young infant is by the mother getting a vaccination near the beginning of the third trimester in every pregnancy. Even if a mother has had a recent booster, it allows extra maternal antibodies to cross the placenta, providing protection for the baby during the time they are most vulnerable: the first six weeks after birth. Boosters are also recommended for adults in close contact with infants.

Newborn visitors and vaccinations

I recommend a whooping cough (pertussis) vaccine booster for anyone spending a lot of time with a newborn, if they have not had a booster in the past ten years. Immunity to whooping cough wanes over time, and it is particularly dangerous for young babies. If you and your family feel strongly about certain vaccines, you have every right to make your own choices. I urge open, courteous conversations around this topic, with a particular focus on a happy, settled baby and a recovering mother.

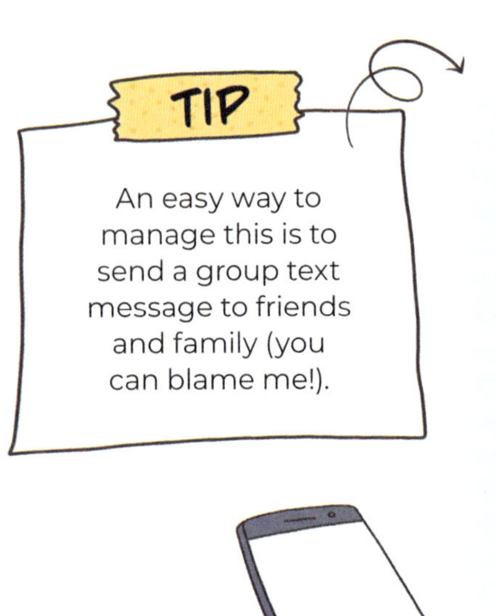

Hi, loved ones! We can't wait to welcome our new baby to the world shortly. We'd love you to come for a cuddle, and our paediatrician has recommended that visitors have their whooping cough vax booster shot if they haven't had a booster in the past ten years. Also, just as a general rule: delay your visit if you've got a cold. Thanks so much!

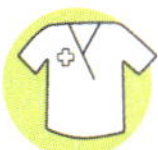

Treatment and management at home

If you suspect your child has whooping cough, contact your local doctor immediately. Early diagnosis and treatment with antibiotics – for both the child and close contacts – can help reduce the severity of symptoms and prevent the spread to others.

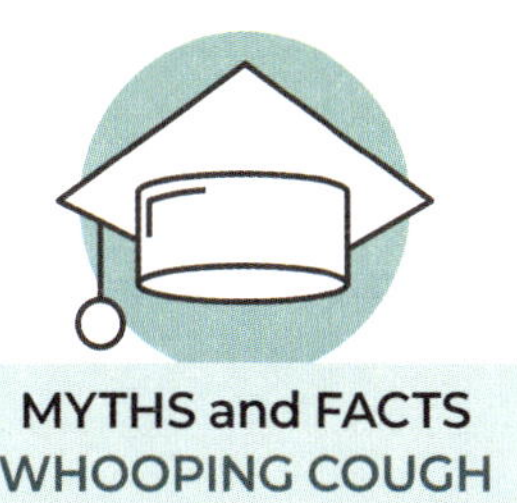

MYTHS and FACTS
WHOOPING COUGH

Myth: Whooping cough only affects babies and young children.

Fact: It's most serious in infants but anyone can get whooping cough. Trust me, it's not fun for an adult to have a cough that lasts 100 days.

Myth: The pertussis vaccine is 100 per cent effective.

Fact: While the vaccine is very effective, it's not perfect – efficacy sits at approximately 85 per cent. Some vaccinated individuals may still get whooping cough, but their illness is usually milder and shorter.

Childcare or school exclusion

For confirmed pertussis, the child should not return to school until they have completed five days of a course of antibiotics targeted to treat pertussis, or for twenty-one days from the beginning of their cough.

Remember: By staying informed and vaccinating your children, you can help protect them from this serious illness.

Upper respiratory illnesses

COVID-19

In the past few years, there has probably been no virus more discussed, researched and worried over than COVID-19. While the weight of the global pandemic has largely shifted, it's still important to understand how COVID-19 affects children, to separate fact from fiction, and to know when to seek medical help for your child.

SYMPTOMS: FEVER, COUGH, RUNNY NOSE, SORE THROAT, FATIGUE, HEADACHE

What is COVID-19?

COVID-19, short for **co**rona**vi**rus **d**isease 20**19**, is caused by a virus called SARS-CoV-2. It primarily affects the respiratory system (nose, throat and lungs), but can also cause symptoms in other parts of the body.

Who does it affect?

COVID-19 can infect people of all ages, including children. However, most children experience milder illness than adults.

How does COVID-19 spread?

COVID-19 spreads easily through respiratory droplets when an infected person coughs or sneezes. It can survive on surfaces for some time, meaning that people can catch it from touching contaminated surfaces and then touching their face, eating or drinking.

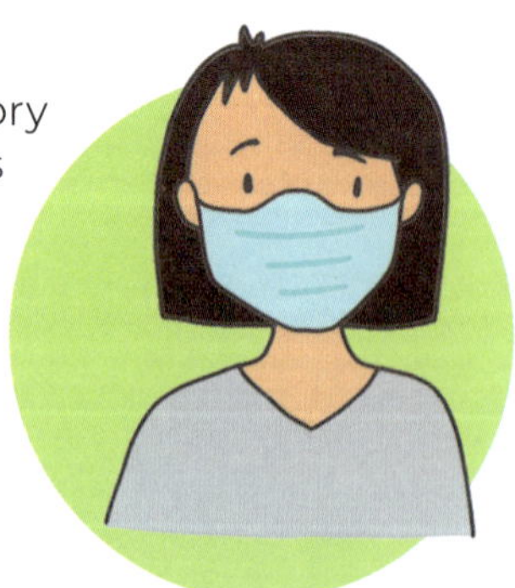

 Recognising the symptoms (in children)

The symptoms of COVID-19 in children can vary widely. The usual symptoms resemble those of the common cold or influenza, including fever, cough, runny nose, sore throat, fatigue and headache. Less commonly, children may experience muscle aches, nausea and vomiting, diarrhoea, loss of taste or smell, shortness of breath, and a rash.

The far less common, but serious, complication of COVID-19 is multi-system inflammatory syndrome in children (MIS-C). This is a rare but serious complication that can occur several weeks after a COVID-19 infection. It can affect multiple organs, can result in significant illness and requires immediate medical attention.

The typical course of COVID-19 in children
Symptoms typically appear two to fourteen days after exposure to the virus. Most children recover within one or two weeks, but some may experience symptoms for longer.

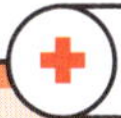 SEEK MEDICAL HELP

Contact your doctor or seek immediate medical care if your child:

- has trouble breathing
- has persistent pain or pressure in the chest
- is confused or difficult to wake up
- has blue lips or face
- has signs of dehydration (dry mouth, no tears, little or no urine)
- has new or worsening symptoms
- has any symptoms that concern you.

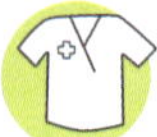 Treatment and management at home

Most children with COVID-19 recover at home with supportive care. This includes plenty of rest, adequate hydration and fever-reducing medications (if needed and as directed by your doctor). COVID-19 is such a recent bug that research is still evolving, with new recommendations appearing regularly. At the time of publication, antiviral medications aren't recommended for most children.

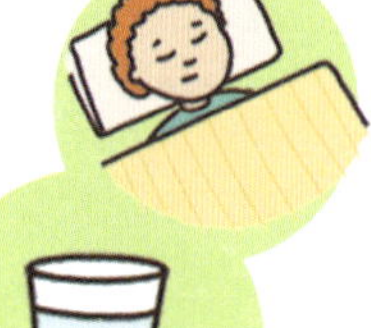

- **Rest:** Lots of it! Let your child sleep as much as they need.
- **Fluids:** Offer water, clear broths, electrolyte drinks and icy poles to keep them hydrated.
- **Fever and pain relief:** Children's paracetamol or ibuprofen can help manage fever and aches.
- **Humidifier:** A cool-mist humidifier can soothe a sore throat and stuffy nose.

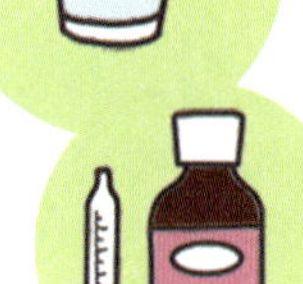

Prevention

The best way to protect your child is through:

1. **Vaccination:** COVID-19 vaccines are safe and effective for children.
2. **Hygiene:** Frequent handwashing, covering coughs and sneezes.
3. **Staying home when sick:** Keep your child home if they have any symptoms of illness.

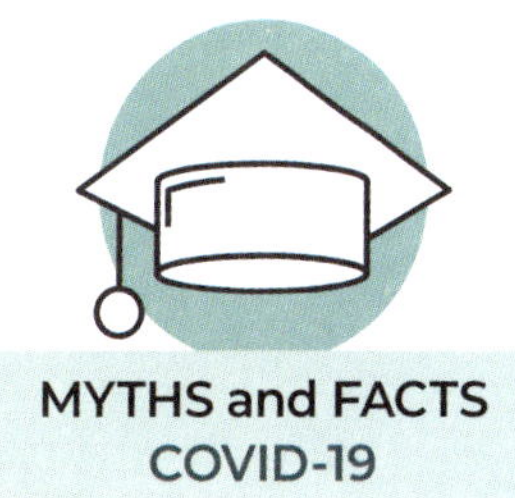

MYTHS and FACTS COVID-19

Myth: Children don't get COVID-19.

Fact: Children can and do get COVID-19, although they are less likely to become severely ill. Most children have mild symptoms or no symptoms at all (asymptomatic).

Myth: COVID-19 is never serious in children.

Fact: While it is rare, some children can develop severe illness, especially those with underlying health conditions.

Childcare or school exclusion

It is best to keep your child home until they are well again.

Remember: If you have any questions or concerns about COVID-19 and your child, please don't hesitate to reach out to your doctor. We're here to help.

Upper respiratory illnesses

Asthma

SYMPTOMS: WHEEZING, COUGHING, SHORTNESS OF BREATH, CHEST TIGHTNESS, NIGHT-TIME AWAKENINGS

What is asthma?

Imagine your child's airways are like little tubes. With asthma, these tubes become sensitive and easily inflamed or swollen, making it harder for air to flow out of the lungs. This leads to the classic symptoms of asthma: wheeze, cough, shortness of breath and chest tightness.

Diving a little deeper, asthma affects the small air passages of the lungs, when a certain trigger causes the airway to produce mucus and narrow too quickly, too easily and too much.

These little airways have an inner lining (called mucosa), surrounded by a muscle (called smooth muscle). When an asthmatic child encounters a trigger, the smooth rings of this muscle tighten, narrowing the air passages. At the same time, the mucosa lining becomes inflamed and releases more mucus, further blocking the air passages.

The mucus itself is normal and healthy; it helps to trap foreign particles like dust and pollen that enter the lungs. But during an asthma attack, there's too much of it, which makes it harder to breathe.

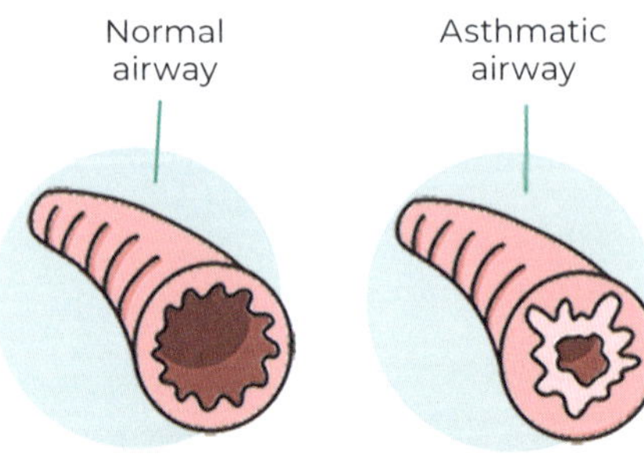

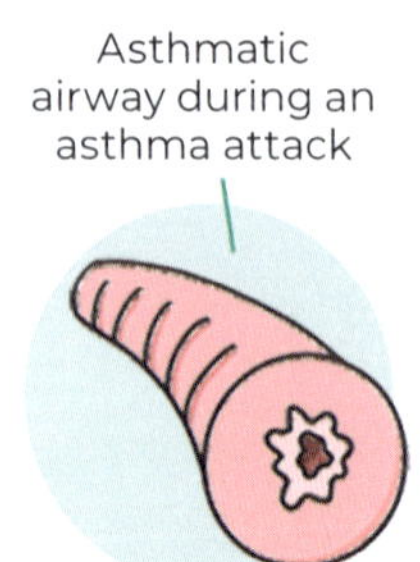

Who is affected by asthma?

Asthma can affect adults and children of all ages, though it's seldom diagnosed under two years. Approximately 20 per cent of children will be diagnosed with asthma during childhood, and many will outgrow this in time. It often runs in families, but sometimes there's no clear cause. The good news is that almost all asthmatic children can lead a normal and active life, with an asthma action plan in place.

FAQ: My eighteen-month-old is wheezing. Is it asthma?

Asthma is complicated in children under two

In children under the age of two, there are many factors which make the diagnosis of asthma difficult:

1. They have smaller airways and less mature immune systems. This means they catch many viruses that cause inflammation and mucus, leading to wheeze. This viral-induced wheeze is not the same as asthma. Many children who have wheeze with recurrent respiratory infections in early infancy do not go on to develop asthma.

2. Because of their immature airways, they do not respond to treatment used for asthma, and trying to do lung function tests is challenging. A lung function test measures how well the lungs work. It's often used to diagnose or monitor lung conditions like asthma. It requires cooperation from the child to do a series of tests, which can be difficult in younger children.

Your doctor or paediatrician will monitor your child if they have persistent symptoms in early infancy or if they have a family history of severe asthma and allergies. Children under two rarely receive a diagnosis of asthma – instead it is labelled as 'viral-induced wheeze' until they are older, when your doctor will have a clearer picture of what's going on.

Recognising the symptoms

Here are some of the telltale signs of asthma in children:

- **Wheezing:** A whistling sound when breathing, especially when breathing out.
- **Coughing:** This can be worse at night or during exercise.
- **Shortness of breath:** Your child might breathe faster than usual or have trouble keeping up with their friends during play.
- **Chest tightness:** They might describe it as a feeling of pressure or squeezing in their chest. Some describe not being able to take a deep breath.
- **Night-time awakenings:** Coughing or difficulty breathing can wake them up. Quite often, a night-time cough is the only presenting symptom of asthma.

Not every child experiences all of these symptoms, and the severity can really vary.

What triggers an asthma attack?

There are many different triggers that can cause a child to have an acute exacerbation of asthma, more colloquially known as an asthma attack.

If your child has asthma or asthma-like symptoms, it's important that you identify their common triggers so that you can do your best to avoid them, or, if unavoidable, you are prepared for an inevitable episode.

Common categories of asthma triggers:

1. changes in season or abrupt weather changes like thunderstorms
2. certain medications
3. inhalation of substances like fire smoke, cigarette smoke, pollens and dust
4. medical allergies or sensitivities, from foods and animals to pollen and grass
5. exercise
6. the common cold or other viruses
7. high emotions, including stress, crying or laughing.

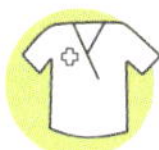 Treatment and management at home

Asthma attacks: what to do

Every child with an asthma diagnosis requires an up-to-date asthma action plan. This should be an easily accessed document, developed together with your child's doctor, so you (or your child's carer, teacher, etc.) know exactly what to do in the event of an asthma attack. The plan usually involves using a reliever inhaler (a puffer used with a spacer) to quickly open the airways. It may also include other medicines (inhaled or oral) to use in the hours and days following an episode.

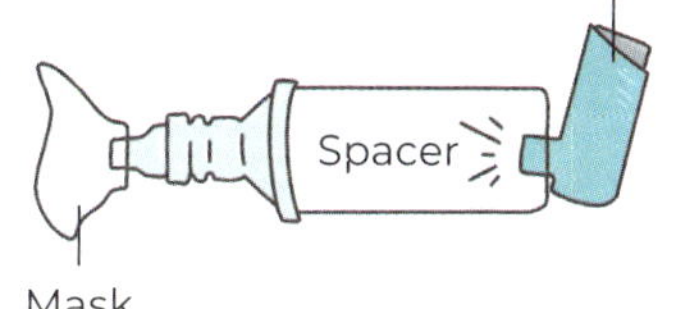

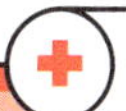

SEEK URGENT MEDICAL HELP

If your child shows any of the following, seek urgent medical attention:

- severe difficulty breathing, or wheezing that doesn't improve with medication
- bluish lips or fingernails
- extreme tiredness or confusion
- inability to speak in full sentences.

Managing asthma: a partnership with your doctor

The good news is that asthma is a manageable condition. Your doctor will work with you to develop a personalised asthma action plan, which might include:

- **Medications:** Preventers (taken daily to reduce inflammation) and relievers (used as needed to open airways during an attack). Sometimes oral medications are also used for brief periods (steroids).
- **Trigger avoidance:** Identifying and avoiding triggers like dust mites, pollen, smoke and pet dander.

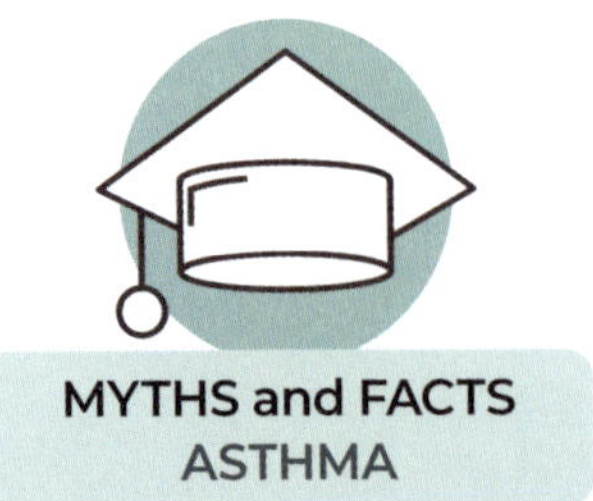

Myth: Kids with asthma can't play sports.

Fact: With proper management, most kids with asthma can be active and participate in all sports. With an asthma action plan and medications readily available, very few asthmatic children have any limitations imposed.

Myth: All asthma medications are the same.

Fact: There are different types of asthma medications, each with a specific purpose. Some are used to prevent symptoms (preventers), while others are used to relieve them (relievers).

Childcare or school exclusion

There is no need to exclude a child with asthma. However, after an asthma attack, return to school when symptoms are resolving and they only require Ventolin once or not at all while at school, on a weaning dose.

Remember: While asthma can be challenging, it doesn't have to define your child's life. With the right knowledge, medications and support, most children with asthma can lead full, active lives.

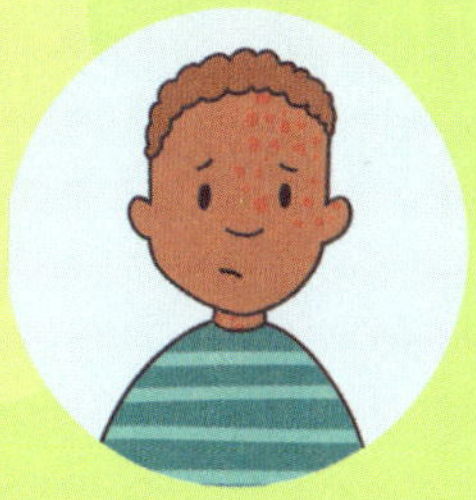

Viruses with rashes

HFMD: hand, foot and mouth disease

I know, the name can sound a bit alarming! Rest assured, this is a very common childhood illness, and most children experience a mild course, recovering without any complications.

SYMPTOMS: MILD FEVER, SORE THROAT, GENERAL DISCOMFORT AND TIREDNESS, PAINFUL ULCERS, RASH ON HANDS, FEET, BOTTOM OR GENITALS

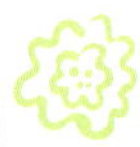

What is HFMD?

HFMD is primarily caused by a virus (usually from the coxsackie group of enteroviruses, most commonly coxsackie virus A16). It's highly contagious and easily spreads from person to person through direct contact with the saliva, nasal mucus or fluid from the blisters of an infected individual. It can also be transmitted through contact with contaminated surfaces or objects.

Who is most at risk of HFMD?

Children under five are most susceptible to HFMD, though older children and adults can also contract the virus. This is *not* the same as foot-and-mouth disease, which affects livestock and can't affect humans.

Recognising the symptoms

The initial symptoms of HFMD often mimic a common cold, with mild fever, sore throat, general discomfort and tiredness. Within a day or two, painful ulcers may develop in the mouth, tongue, gums or inner cheeks. This can make eating and drinking uncomfortable. Around the same time, or shortly after, a rash may appear on the hands, feet, and sometimes the bottom or genitals. This rash typically consists of red spots or blisters that are not usually itchy.

Ulcers:

This is the first sign, and that which childcare or school staff will look for to quickly identify HFMD.

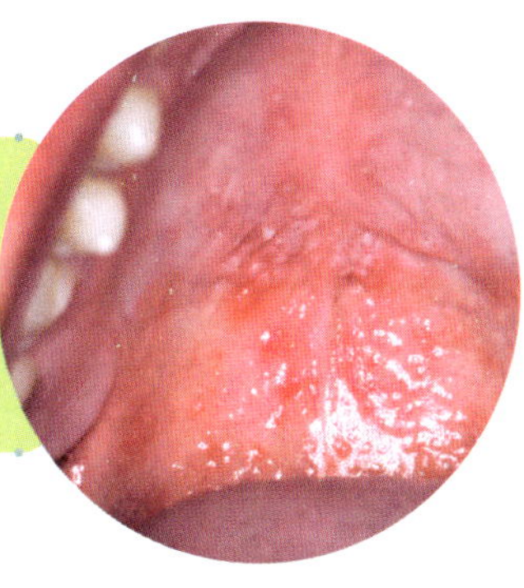

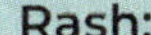

Rash:

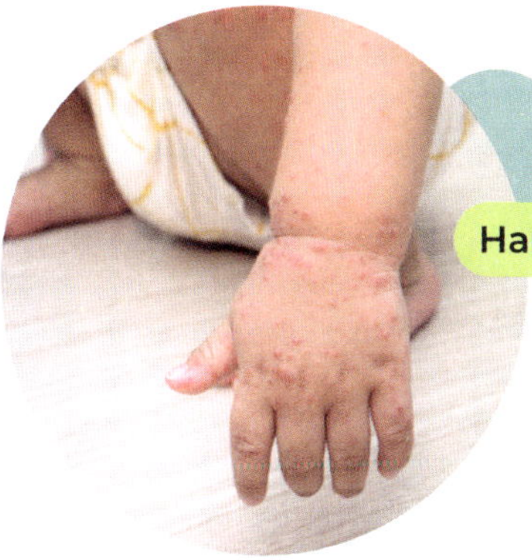

Hand

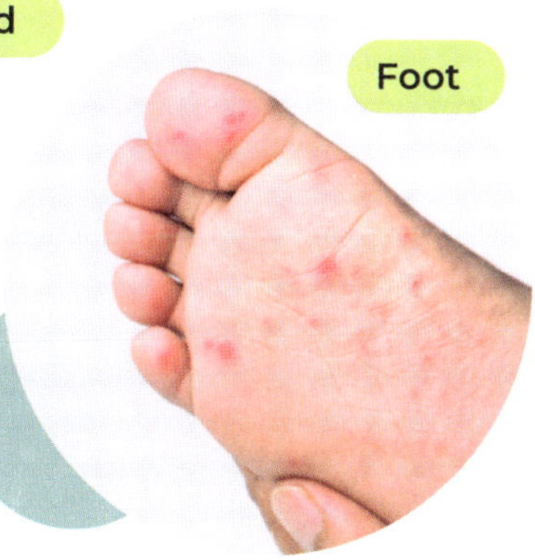

Foot

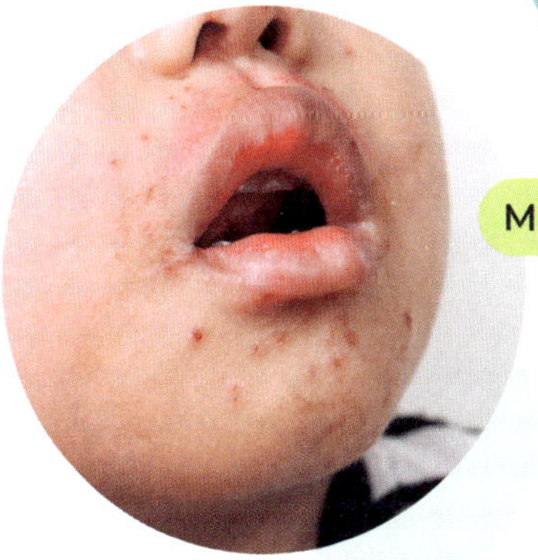

Mouth

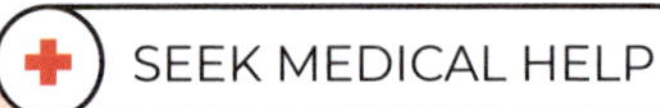

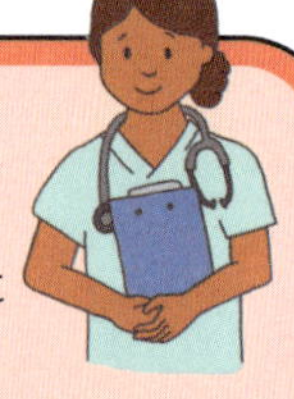

Most cases of HFMD are mild and can be managed at home. However, you should consult your doctor if:

- your child is under three months old and has a fever
- your child seems very unwell or drowsy or is difficult to wake up
- your child has fewer wet nappies or is showing signs of dehydration (dry mouth, sunken eyes, no tears when crying)
- the rash appears infected (red, swollen or oozing pus)
- your child has a weakened immune system.

The typical course of HFMD

HFMD usually runs its course within seven to ten days. Your child is most contagious during the first week of illness, but the virus can continue to be shed in poo for several weeks after recovery. This means it's important to maintain good hygiene practices, such as thorough handwashing, to prevent the spread of the virus. Once your child has recovered, don't be alarmed if affected skin peels off in the following weeks. If, however, you notice skin peeling and your child is still unwell, have them reviewed by a doctor.

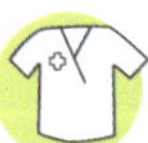

Treatment and management at home

There is no specific treatment for HFMD, as it's a viral infection that typically resolves on its own, but you can focus on providing your child with comfort and relief from their symptoms.

- **Pain relief:** Over-the-counter medications like paracetamol or ibuprofen can help manage fever and discomfort. Always follow the recommended dosage for your child's age and weight.
- **Fluids:** Encourage your child to drink plenty of fluids, such as water, or breastmilk or formula for infants. This will help prevent dehydration, especially if they have a sore throat or fever.

The painful mouth ulcers with HFMD can often inhibit drinking so much that children become dangerously dehydrated. Don't hesitate to see your doctor if this is happening with your child.

- **Soft foods:** Offer soft, bland foods that are easy to swallow, such as yoghurt, apple puree or soup. Avoid acidic or spicy foods, as these can irritate mouth sores.

Prevention

To reduce the risk of your child getting or spreading HFMD, practise good hygiene habits, such as frequent handwashing, especially after changing nappies or using the toilet. Teach your child to cover their mouth and nose when coughing or sneezing, and disinfect frequently touched surfaces and toys regularly.

Many people think that if they've had HFMD once, they are immune for life, but because it can be caused by a number of different viruses, you can absolutely contract HFMD more than once.

Childcare or school exclusion

Your child should remain home until all the blisters have dried to prevent further transmission of infection.

Remember: HFMD is a common childhood illness with a generally favourable course. By recognising the symptoms, providing supportive care, and seeking medical advice when needed, you can ensure your child is comfortable and has a speedy recovery.

If you have any further questions or concerns, don't hesitate to reach out to your paediatrician. We're here to support you and your child's health journey.

Viruses with rashes

Chickenpox

Chickenpox is a common childhood illness that's known for its itchy, blister-like rash. While it can be a bit of a nuisance, it's usually a mild illness that runs its course without complications. There are lots of things you can do to help your little one feel more comfortable while they recover.

SYMPTOMS: ITCHY RASH OF RED BUMPS AND BLISTERS, FEVER, HEADACHE, FATIGUE, LOSS OF APPETITE

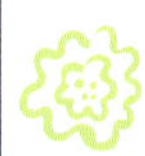

What is chickenpox?

Chickenpox is a highly contagious viral infection caused by the varicella-zoster virus (VZV). It's most common in children under twelve, but it can occur at any age. The virus spreads easily through the air when an infected person coughs or sneezes, or through direct contact with the fluid from the blisters. Rates of chickenpox infection have decreased dramatically since the introduction of the VZV vaccine.

Recognising the symptoms

The hallmark symptom of chickenpox is the itchy rash that starts as small red bumps and quickly turns into fluid-filled blisters. These blisters then break open, crust over and eventually heal. The rash usually begins on the chest, back and face, and then spreads to the rest of the body.

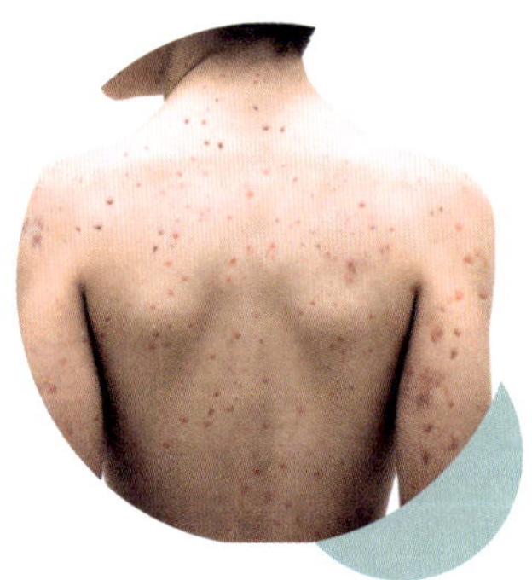

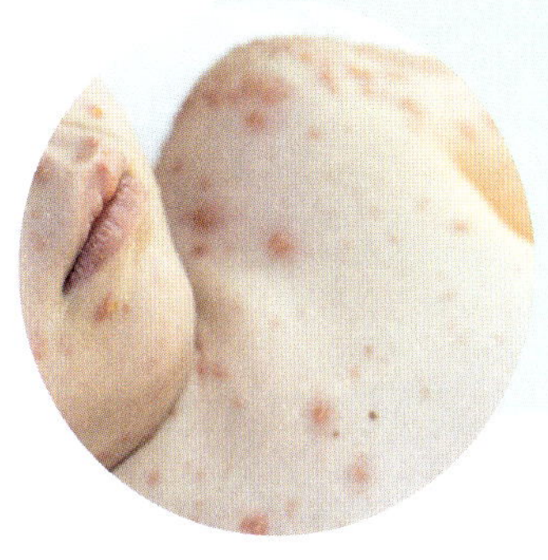

Besides the rash, your child might also experience:

- **Fever:** A low-grade fever is common, but it can sometimes be higher.
- **Headache:** Often mild to moderate in intensity.

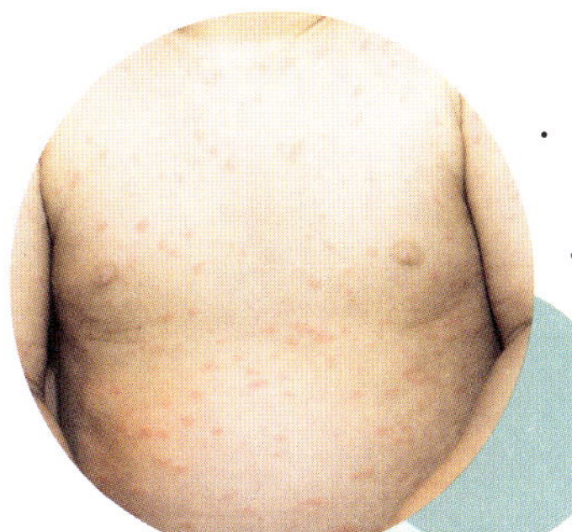

- **Fatigue:** Your child may feel tired and lack energy.
- **Loss of appetite:** Your child may not feel like eating as much as usual.

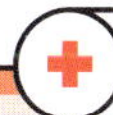

SEEK MEDICAL HELP

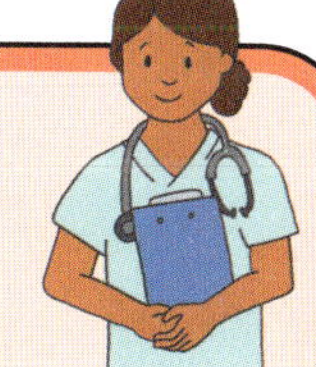

Most cases of chickenpox are mild, but it's important to seek medical advice if:

- your child is less than twelve months old
- your child has a weakened immune system
- your child's fever is high (above 38.5°C) and lasts for more than a few days
- your child has difficulty breathing or a severe cough
- the rash looks infected (red, swollen or oozing pus)
- you have any concerns about your child's condition
- if your child develops a red eye 'conjunctivitis' during the course of the illness. They may also complain of eye pain, sensitivity to light, tearing and blurred vision.

The typical course of chickenpox

Chickenpox typically lasts for seven to ten days. Your child is most contagious from one to two days *before* the rash appears until all the blisters have crusted over. It's important to keep them home from school or childcare during this time to prevent spreading the virus to others.

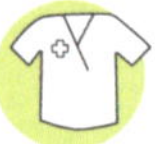

Treatment and management at home

While a vaccine exists, there's no cure for chickenpox, but there are plenty of ways to manage the symptoms and make your child more comfortable:

- **Soothe the itch:** Calamine lotion, oatmeal baths, antihistamines and cool compresses can help relieve itching.
- **Pain relief:** Over-the-counter medications like paracetamol or ibuprofen can help with fever and discomfort.
- **Prevent scratching:** Keep your child's fingernails short to prevent scratching, which can lead to infection and scarring.
- **Hydration:** Encourage your child to drink plenty of fluids to prevent dehydration.
- **Rest:** Make sure your child gets plenty of rest, as their body needs energy to fight off the virus.

Prevention

The best way to prevent chickenpox is through vaccination. The chickenpox vaccine is safe and effective, and it's recommended for all children as part of their routine immunisation schedule. While 'chickenpox parties' used to be all the rage a generation ago, they are definitely not recommended now.

A note on shingles

Shingles is the sneaky sequel to chickenpox. The VZV that causes chickenpox sometimes reappears later in life as shingles, no matter when – or how severe – the original infection was. Reactivation of VZV causes a painful, blistering rash, usually on one side of the body. Think of it like this: the chickenpox virus takes a long nap in your nervous system after you've had chickenpox, and sometimes, it wakes up grumpy and causes shingles.

While there's no cure for shingles, there are ways to manage it and reduce the discomfort. Antiviral medications can help shorten the illness and prevent complications. Pain relief is also important, and your doctor might recommend over-the-counter options or prescription medications depending on the severity.

Cooling compresses and calamine lotion can soothe the skin, and rest is crucial for recovery. As with chickenpox, if you become concerned about eye infection, you should seek immediate medical review.

Childcare or school exclusion

Your child should remain home until all the blisters have dried, which is usually around five days after the rash first appears, to prevent further transmission of infection. If your child was at school the day or so prior to rash development, it is important to notify the school of your child's diagnosis.

Remember: Chickenpox is a common childhood illness, and most children recover without complications. By understanding the symptoms and providing supportive care, you can help your child navigate through the itchy phase and emerge with a new-found immunity.

If you have any further questions or concerns, don't hesitate to reach out to your local doctor. We're here to support you and your child on their health journey.

Viruses with rashes

Slapped cheek

Slapped cheek can seem like a bizarre condition. It's usually very mild, but its appearance – and rapidity of onset – can make it very alarming for parents and caregivers. Beyond the uncomfortable colloquial term, it is also called fifth disease or erythema infectiosum.

SYMPTOMS: MILD FEVER, RUNNY NOSE, SORE THROAT, HEADACHE, NAUSEA, RASH ON CHEEKS AND BODY

What is slapped cheek?

Slapped cheek is caused by a virus called parvovirus B19. It's most common in children between four and ten years but can affect people of all ages. This virus is pretty sneaky – it often starts with mild cold-like symptoms, and by the time the signature rash appears on your child's cheeks, they might not even feel sick anymore!

Recognising the symptoms

The first signs (most infectious during this period):

- **Mild fever:** Children will commonly get a low-grade fever before the rash.
- **Runny nose, sore throat, headache:** Think 'common cold' symptoms.
- **Upset stomach, feeling generally unwell:** Your child might be a little queasy or just feel generally off.

A few days into the illness:

- **Bright red rash on the cheeks:** This is the hallmark sign, making it look like someone gave your child a light slap. This usually occurs as the fever breaks.

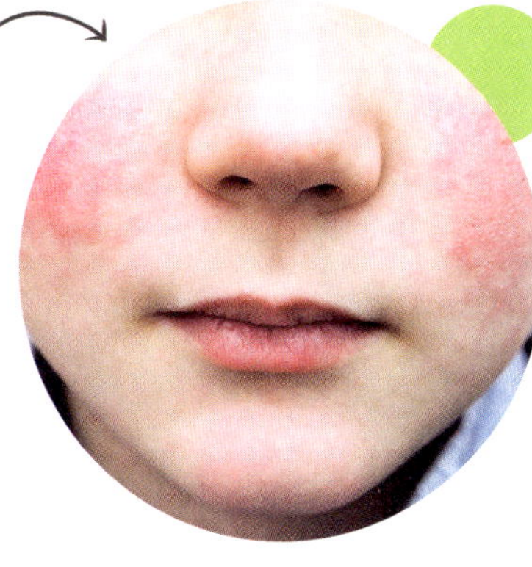

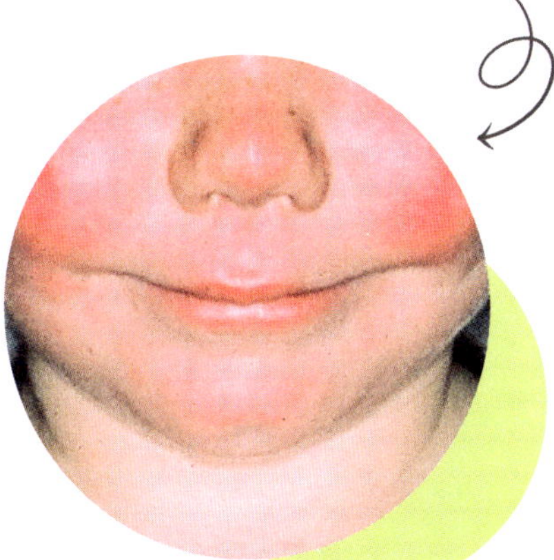

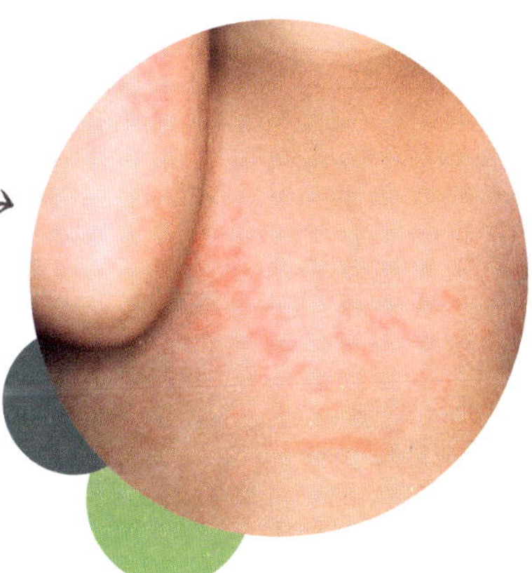

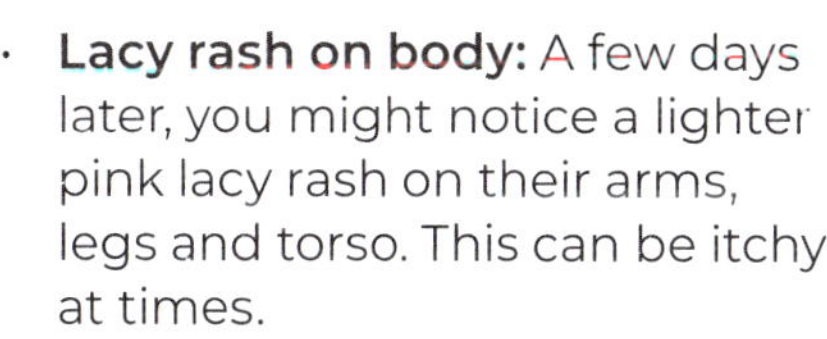

- **Lacy rash on body:** A few days later, you might notice a lighter pink lacy rash on their arms, legs and torso. This can be itchy at times.

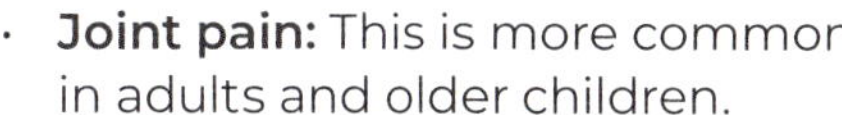

- **Joint pain:** This is more common in adults and older children.

The typical course of slapped cheek

The good news is that slapped cheek usually runs its course within a week or two. The facial rash fades first, but the body rash can come and go for a few weeks, especially if your child gets hot or spends time in the sun.

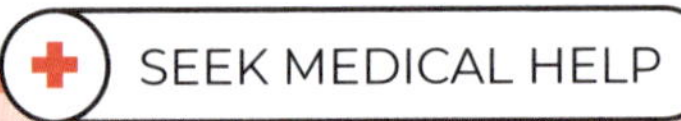

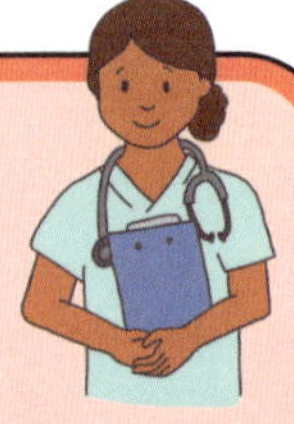

Most of the time, slapped cheek is nothing to worry about. But here's when you should call your doctor:

1. **Your child has a weakened immune system:** Kids with certain health conditions might need closer monitoring.
2. **Severe symptoms:** High fever that doesn't come down, difficulty breathing or extreme fatigue warrant a call.
3. **You're pregnant and exposed:** The virus can be more serious for pregnant women, so let your doctor know if you've been exposed to someone with slapped cheek. If your child has had slapped cheek, notify any contacts of yours who may be pregnant.

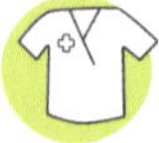

Treatment and management at home

Because it's a virus, there's no specific medicine to treat slapped cheek. Here's what you can do at home:

- **Rest:** Let your child rest as much as they need to.
- **Fluids:** Offer plenty of water and other clear liquids.
- **Fever and pain relief:** If your child has a fever or aches, children's paracetamol or ibuprofen can help.
- **Soothe the rash:** A cool compress, antihistamines or calamine lotion can help with itching.

Protecting others: preventing the spread

Since slapped cheek is contagious, here are some easy ways to reduce the spread:

- **Handwashing:** Teach your kids to wash their hands often (and lead by example!).
- **Cover coughs and sneezes:** Encourage your child to use a tissue or elbow.
- **Don't share:** Avoid sharing utensils, cups or towels.

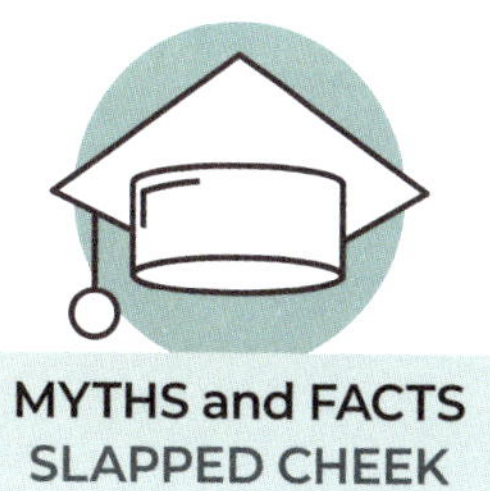

MYTHS and FACTS
SLAPPED CHEEK

Myth: Slapped cheek is always serious.

Fact: Most kids have very mild symptoms and recover without any issues.

Myth: You can get slapped cheek multiple times.

Fact: Once you've had it, you're immune for life.

Myth: All kids get the 'slapped cheek' rash.

Fact: Some kids only have a body rash or mild cold symptoms. This is why some people don't realise they've had parvovirus B19 infection.

Childcare or school exclusion

Your child does not need to be excluded from school or daycare so long as they are twenty-four hours fever-free. Once the rash appears they are no longer infectious. You should let the school know, however, so that other families can be made aware, as it is a risk to non-immune pregnant women.

Remember: While it can be startling to see your child's face turn bright red, remember that slapped cheek is usually a mild and temporary illness. With rest, fluids and a little TLC, your child will be back to their usual self in no time. As always, if you have any concerns, don't hesitate to reach out to your local doctor. We're here to help!

Cold sores

Ah, cold sores – those tiny, fluid-filled blisters that seem to pop up at the most inconvenient times. If you have ever experienced a cold sore, you know how uncomfortable they can be. I often get questions about cold sores in children, so let's break down what they are, why they happen and how to manage them.

SYMPTOMS: TINGLING OR BURNING SKIN AROUND THE MOUTH, SMALL, PAINFUL BLISTERS ON LIPS OR MOUTH

What are cold sores?

Cold sores are small, painful blisters that usually appear on the lips or around the mouth. They're caused by herpes simplex virus type 1 (HSV-1), a very common virus that most people are exposed to at some point in their lives. Don't let the name fool you – cold sores aren't actually related to colds.

Why do kids get cold sores?

Kids can catch HSV-1 through direct contact with someone who has a cold sore or by sharing drink bottles, cutlery, towels or other items. Many children get their first infection during their preschool years, and it often goes unnoticed or they have very mild symptoms. Some children – thankfully rarely – can have a significant outbreak in their first episode, leading to painful blisters that make swallowing nearly impossible. This is a major red flag for dehydration, and these children MUST be reviewed by your local doctor or emergency department.

The typical course of a cold sore

Cold sores typically heal within seven to ten days. The good news is that the first outbreak is usually the worst. Subsequent outbreaks tend to be milder and less frequent.

Recognising the symptoms

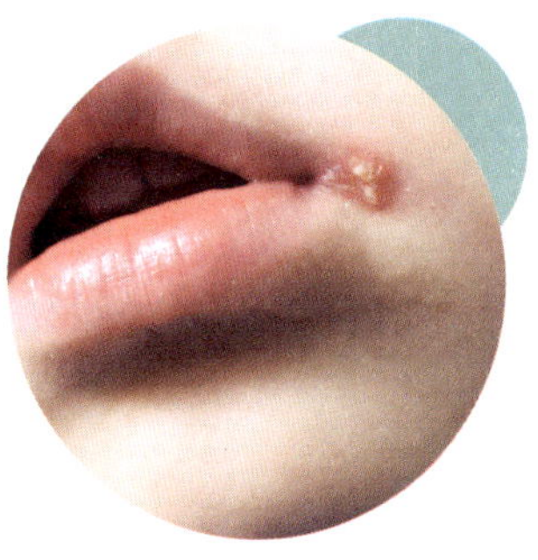

1. **Tingling or burning skin:** Before the blister appears, your child might report feeling a tingling, itching or burning sensation around their mouth.

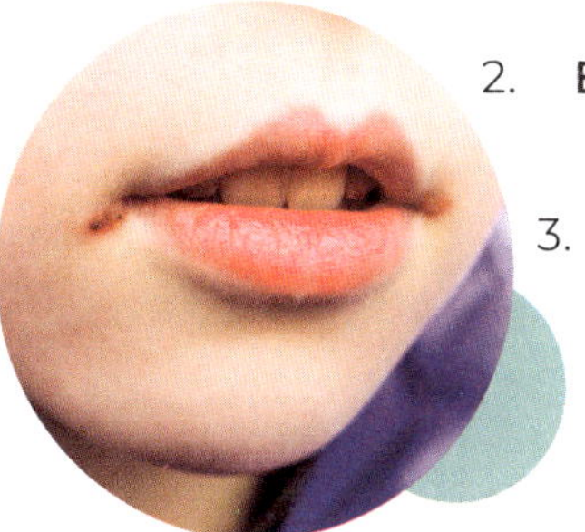

2. **Blister formation:** Small, painful blisters will then develop, usually on the lips.
3. **Oozing and crusting:** The blisters may break open, ooze and then form a yellowish crust.

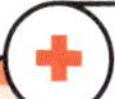

SEEK MEDICAL HELP

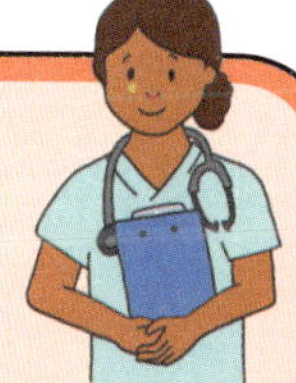

Most cold sores can be managed at home, but you should consult your local doctor if:

- your child is under six months old
- the cold sore is very large or painful
- your child has a fever or other signs of illness
- the cold sore doesn't heal within ten days
- there is a newborn around
- if your child has recurrent cold sore outbreaks. An antiviral medication may be needed to reduce the frequency of outbreaks.

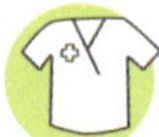

Treatment and management at home

Though there's no cure for cold sores, there are things you can do to ease your child's discomfort and speed up healing:

- **Over-the-counter creams:** These may help reduce the duration of the cold sore. Lip balms aren't recommended as they can inadvertently spread the virus.
- **Prescription medications:** In some cases, your local doctor might prescribe an antiviral cream or oral medication, especially for severe or frequent outbreaks.
- **Pain relief:** Over-the-counter pain relievers like paracetamol or ibuprofen can help manage any pain, fever or discomfort with eating or drinking.
- **Cold compresses:** Applying a cool, damp cloth to the area can help soothe discomfort.
- **Avoid acidic foods:** Acidic foods like citrus fruits and tomatoes can irritate the sores, so it's best to avoid them while the cold sore is healing.

Protecting others: preventing the spread

Cold sores are contagious, especially when the blisters are oozing. Here are some tips to help prevent the spread:

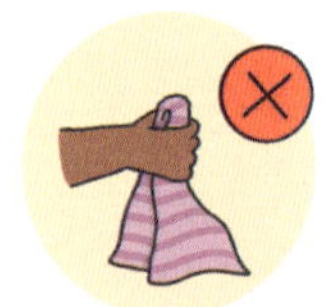

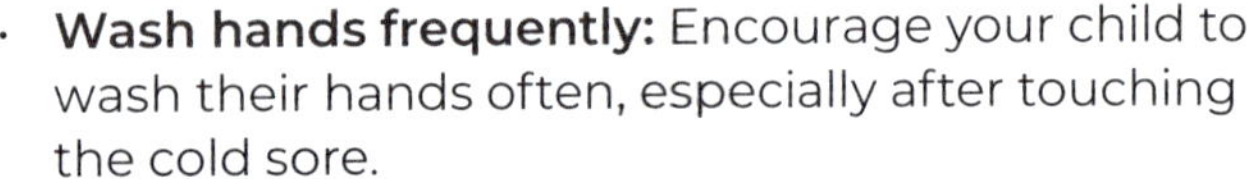

- **Wash hands frequently:** Encourage your child to wash their hands often, especially after touching the cold sore.
- **Don't share:** Avoid sharing utensils, cups, towels or other personal items with your child when they have a cold sore.
- **Don't touch:** Teach your child not to touch or pick at the cold sore.
- **Kissing:** Avoid kissing your child on or near the mouth when they have a cold sore.

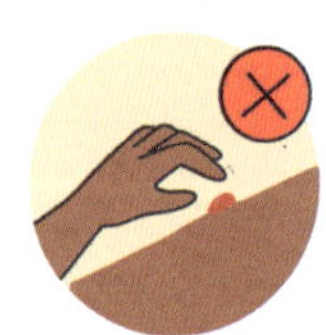

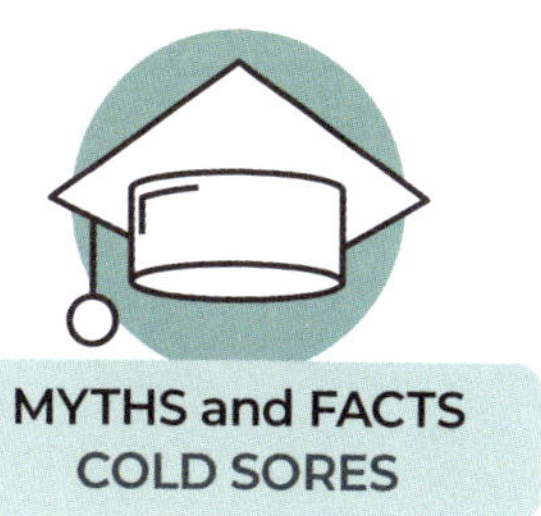

MYTHS and FACTS COLD SORES

Myth: Cold sores are caused by the common cold.

Fact: Cold sores are caused by the herpes simplex virus, not the viruses responsible for the common cold. However, a cold can sometimes trigger a cold sore outbreak due to body stress.

Myth: You can only get cold sores once.

Fact: Unfortunately, once you're infected with HSV-1, the virus remains dormant in your body and can reactivate multiple times, most commonly in times of physical or emotional stress.

Myth: You can get rid of cold sores permanently.

Fact: There's no cure for HSV-1, so cold sores can recur. However, there are treatments to manage outbreaks and reduce their frequency.

Myth: Cold sores are only contagious when the blisters are visible.

Fact: Cold sores are most contagious when they're blistering and oozing, but the virus can still be spread even before the sores appear and after they've crusted over. Many people shed the virus without symptoms. This is why it is best to minimise sharing of drink bottles and utensils where possible.

Childcare or school exclusion

If your child is young and cannot maintain good hygiene practices, then it is best to keep them home while the lesion is weeping. Wherever possible, the lesion should be covered with a dressing.

Remember: Cold sores are a common childhood annoyance, but with a bit of care and attention, you can help your child manage them and prevent spread to others.

Viruses with rashes

Measles

Thanks to vaccination, we've seen measles rates plummet in the space of a single generation. Despite the availability of a vaccine measles outbreaks continue to cause distress in communities around the world. It's important to understand the signs, symptoms and potential complications of this highly contagious disease to ensure your child's health in the event of an outbreak.

SYMPTOMS: HIGH FEVER; COUGH; RUNNY NOSE; RED, WATERY EYES (CONJUNCTIVITIS); KOPLIK SPOTS, FATIQUE, RASH

What are measles?

Measles, also known as rubeola, is a highly contagious viral infection that can cause serious complications, especially in young children. Before the introduction of the measles vaccine, it was a common childhood illness that, sadly, resulted in many deaths worldwide.

How does measles spread?

Measles is incredibly contagious. The virus spreads through the air when an infected person coughs or sneezes. It can linger in the air for up to two hours after the person leaves the room. This means that even brief contact with an infected person can lead to transmission, which is why contact tracing after a confirmed case is so important to limit outbreaks.

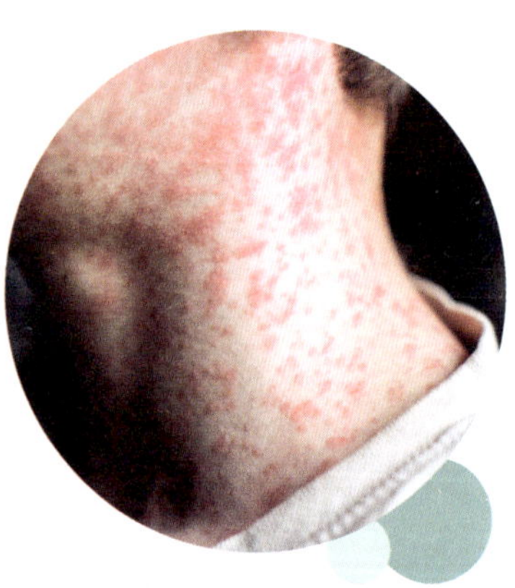

After exposure, symptoms typically take ten to twelve days to appear.

Recognising the symptoms

While the characteristic measles rash is well known, other symptoms often appear first. Here are the signs of measles:

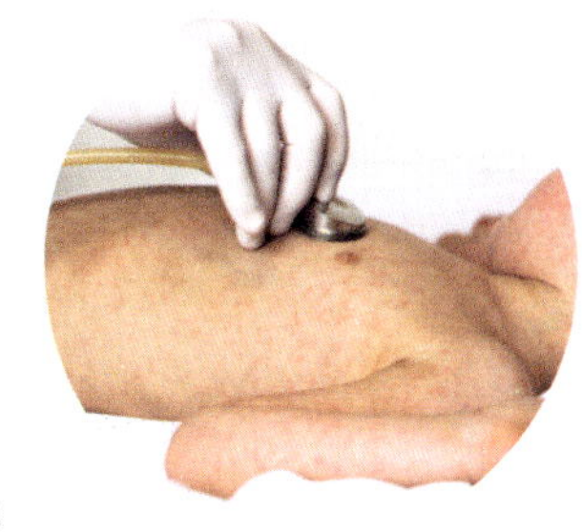

- **High fever:** This can reach 40°C or higher and may last for several days.
- **Cough:** A dry, hacking cough is common.
- **Runny nose:** Similar to a cold.
- **Red, watery eyes (conjunctivitis):** This can cause sensitivity to light.
- **Koplik spots:** These are tiny white spots with bluish-white centres that appear inside the mouth a few days before the rash.
- **Fatigue:** Often feel very tired and exhausted.
- **Rash:** The classic measles rash has a very distinctive pattern of behaviour – it usually starts on the face and spreads downward to the neck, trunk, arms and legs. It typically appears as flat red spots that may eventually merge.

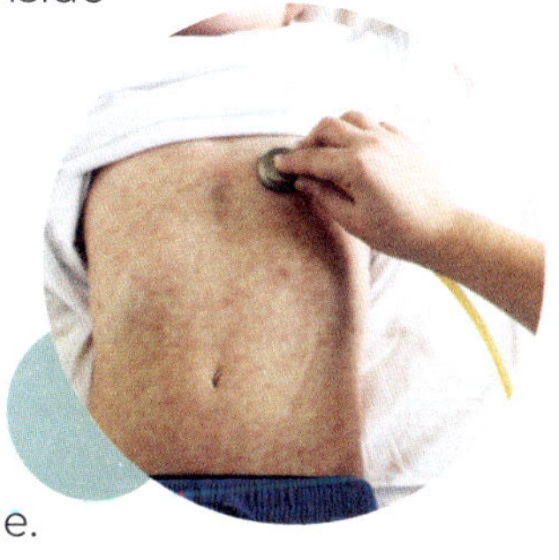

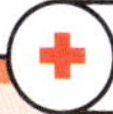

SEEK MEDICAL HELP

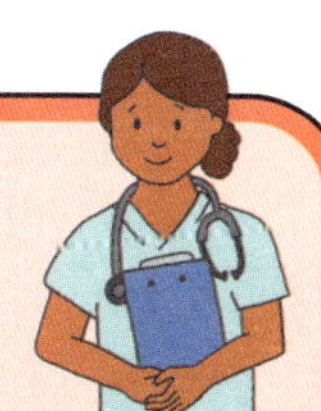

Contact your local doctor immediately if your child:

- has a high fever that doesn't respond to medication
- has difficulty breathing or shows signs of respiratory distress
- develops a stiff neck, seizure or other neurological symptoms
- shows signs of dehydration.

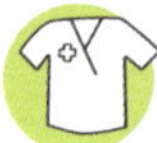

Treatment and management at home

There's no cure for measles, but doctors may consider administering a vaccine or immunoglobulin (blood product) to confirmed cases or contacts. Beyond this, you can help your child recover with:

- **Rest:** Ensure your child gets plenty of rest.
- **Fluids:** Offer plenty of fluids to prevent dehydration.
- **Fever reducers:** Paracetamol or ibuprofen can help manage fever and discomfort.
- **Humidifiers:** A cool-mist humidifier can soothe a cough and sore throat.

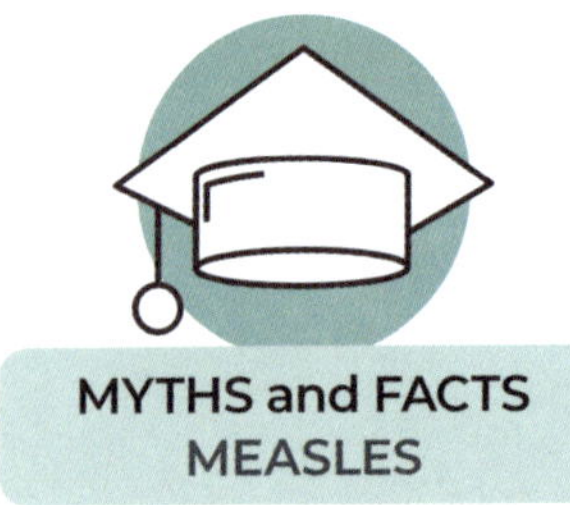

Myth: There's no treatment for measles.

Fact: While there's no specific antiviral medication for measles, supportive care and vitamin A supplementation (in areas where vitamin A deficiency is common) can help reduce the risk of complications.

Myth: Measles is a harmless childhood rash, like chickenpox.

Fact: Measles has the potential to cause serious complications, including pneumonia, encephalitis (brain swelling) and even death.

Prevention: the power of vaccination

The measles, mumps and rubella (MMR) vaccine is the most effective way to protect your child from measles. The vaccine is safe and highly effective, and it's recommended that children receive two doses: the first at twelve months of age and the second between four and six years. Contracting measles, also leads to lifelong immunity.

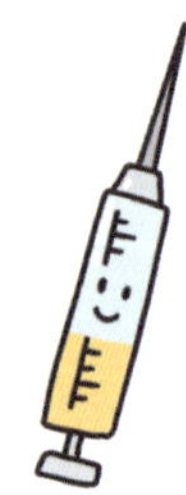

If you have been in contact with someone who is diagnosed with measles, and you are well, it is still worth discussing with your doctor if your child is less than six months of age, or if anyone has a significantly weakened immune system, as a special blood product (immunoglobulin) can be given to confirmed contacts.

Protecting others: isolation is key

If your child develops measles, it's important to keep them isolated from others to prevent spreading the virus. Every local area has different guidelines but, generally, children with measles should stay at home from when symptoms first begin until at least four days after the rash appears. Confirmed contacts who are immunised do not need to be isolated, but unimmunised contacts should stay home for fourteen days after the rash first appears on the initial measles patient.

Measles can be especially harmful for pregnant women, so if you are pregnant and you suspect you've been exposed, discuss it with your doctor. If you think that you have measles, **DO NOT** attend your local doctor or ED without calling ahead to notify them. As measles is extremely contagious, precautions are taken in healthcare settings, such as a separate waiting room.

Childcare or school exclusion

Cases are excluded from school and childcare for at least four days after the rash onset. Immunised contacts are not excluded. Unimmunised contacts should be excluded until fourteen days after the first day of appearance of the rash in the last case. If unimmunised contacts are vaccinated within seventy-two hours of their first contact with the first case, or if they receive immunoglobulin within six days (144 hours) of the contact, they may return to school.

During an outbreak, children and their siblings who are aged from one year to eighteen months should receive their routine second dose of measles-containing vaccine early (but not less than four weeks after their first dose). Guidelines differ across states.

Remember: Measles is a serious illness, but vaccination is the best way to protect your child. If you have any concerns about measles or the vaccine, talk to your local doctor. We're here to help.

Meningococcal disease

Meningococcal disease is a rare but potentially devastating infection that can affect children of all ages. While it can be frightening, full and rapid recovery is the most common outcome, but early recognition and prompt treatment are essential.

SYMPTOMS: SUDDEN HIGH FEVER, SEVERE HEADACHE, STIFF NECK, SENSITIVITY TO LIGHT, NAUSEA AND VOMITING, CONFUSION OR DROWSINESS, RASH

What is meningococcal disease?

Meningococcal disease is a serious bacterial infection caused by the bacterium *Neisseria meningitidis*. It can cause two major illnesses: meningitis (inflammation of the membranes surrounding the brain and spinal cord) and septicaemia (blood poisoning).

How does meningococcal disease spread?

The bacteria spread through close contact with respiratory and throat secretions (saliva) from an infected person. Activities like coughing, kissing and sharing utensils or drinks can transmit the bacteria.

Who is most at risk of meningococcal disease?

While anyone can get meningococcal disease, certain groups are at higher risk: infants and young children under five years old, teenagers and young adults (fifteen to twenty-four years old), those with weakened immune systems and those living in close quarters (e.g. boarding houses, university or college dorms, military barracks).

Recognising the signs: act fast!

I am always loath to raise parents' anxiety levels; you'll more often find me downplaying the need for fear within the parenting sphere. However, meningococcal disease is one condition that can develop rapidly, with potentially catastrophic consequences. It's crucial to recognise the signs and seek medical attention immediately.

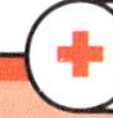

SEEK URGENT MEDICAL HELP

If you suspect meningococcal disease: don't wait! Seek immediate medical attention if your child exhibits any of the symptoms mentioned below. Early diagnosis and treatment are critical for the best possible outcome.

Symptoms of meningococcal disease

- **Sudden high fever:** A fever that comes on quickly and doesn't respond to over-the-counter medications.
- **Leg pain, cold extremities and abnormal skin colour:** If your child has fevers and complains of unexplained calf pain, this should be reviewed by a doctor.
- **Rash:** A rash may appear anywhere on the body, often starting as small red or purple spots that quickly develop into larger, darker patches.

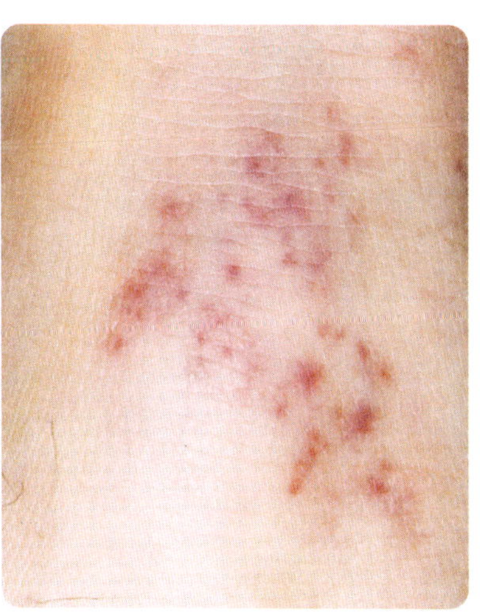

An important note: The rash associated with meningococcal disease doesn't always fade (blanch) when pressed (as some other rashes do). One handy trick is to take clear glass, press it to the rash and look through the glass wall – if the rash disappears, this is a blanching, less concerning rash. A non-blanching rash significantly raises the possibility of meningococcal disease.

Symptoms of meningococcal meningitis:

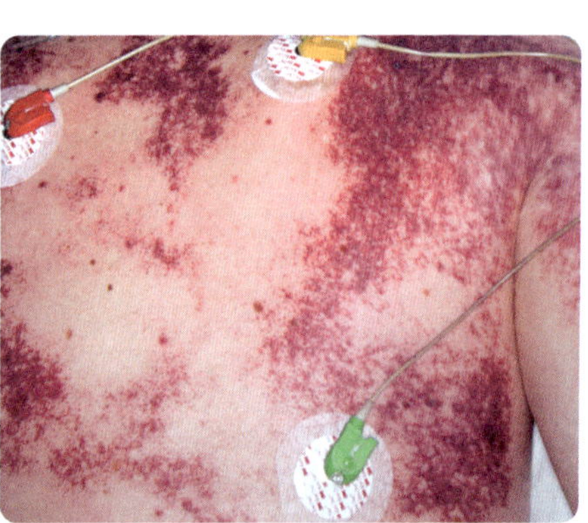

- **Severe headache:** It is often described as the worst headache of someone's life.
- **Stiff neck:** Your child might have difficulty moving the neck or chin towards the chest.
- **Sensitivity to light:** Your child might have discomfort or pain when exposed to bright light.
- **Nausea and vomiting:** These may occur along with the other symptoms.
- **Confusion or drowsiness:** Changes in mental state can indicate a serious infection.

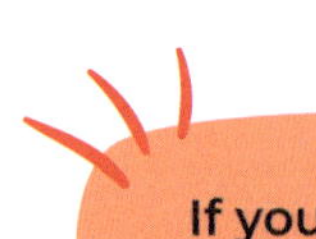

If you suspect meningococcal disease, don't delay seeking medical help.

Prevention: vaccination is key

The good news is that we have safe and effective vaccines to protect against most types of meningococcal bacteria. The Australian National Immunisation Program (NIP) offers free meningococcal vaccines for certain age groups. There are multiple strains, however, including A, B, C, W and Y. Some vaccines are included free for children; others need to be purchased privately. Talk to your doctor to ensure your child is up to date on their vaccinations.

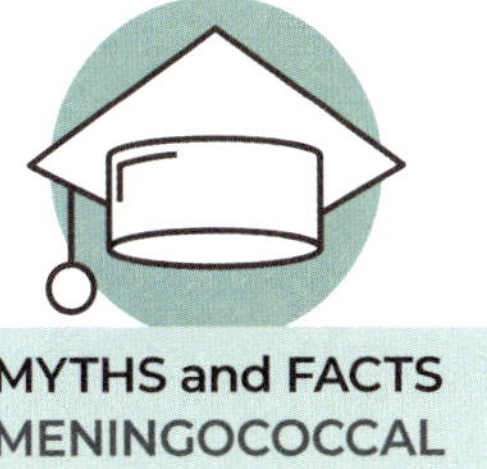

MYTHS and FACTS MENINGOCOCCAL

Myth: Meningococcal disease is always fatal.

Fact: While it can be very serious, with prompt treatment most people recover fully.

Myth: You can't catch meningococcal disease from someone who's vaccinated.

Fact: The vaccine is not 100 per cent effective, so it's still possible, although less likely, to get the disease after vaccination, and to pass it on to others.

Childcare or school exclusion

Children with confirmed meningococcal disease will usually be in hospital during their infectious period. After twenty-four hours of appropriate antibiotic treatment, they will be released from infection control precautions within the hospital. By the time they have left the hospital they should be okay to return to school or childcare. It would be best to check with the treating doctor, though, for specific circumstances.

HSP: Henoch-Schönlein purpura

HSP is caused by inflammation in the small blood vessels of the skin, joints, gut and kidneys. It's most common in children under ten years, though it can occur in adults too. It is not common, occuring in only 0.02 per cent of children.

SYMPTOMS: RASH, JOINT PAIN AND SWELLING, ABDOMINAL PAIN, KIDNEY PROBLEMS

What is HSP?

HSP, also known as IgA vasculitis, is a condition that causes inflammation of the small blood vessels in the body. This swelling can affect various organs, most commonly the skin, joints, intestines and kidneys. While it might sound alarming, the good news is that most children recover from HSP fully, without any long-term complications.

Why does HSP happen?

The exact cause of HSP remains a mystery, but it's often triggered by an infection, such as a cold or the flu. The body's immune system, in its effort to fight off the infection, mistakenly attacks the small blood vessels, leading to inflammation. It's important to note that HSP is not contagious, so your child can't catch it or spread it to others.

Recognising the symptoms

HSP can manifest in various ways, and the most common signs and symptoms include:

- **Rash:** A hallmark of HSP is a characteristic rash that often appears as small red or purple dots or bruises (purpura). This rash typically starts on the lower legs and bottom but can spread to the arms, trunk and face. This rash is commonly mistaken for meningococcal disease, but this should always be decided by a healthcare professional – don't try to diagnose it at home.

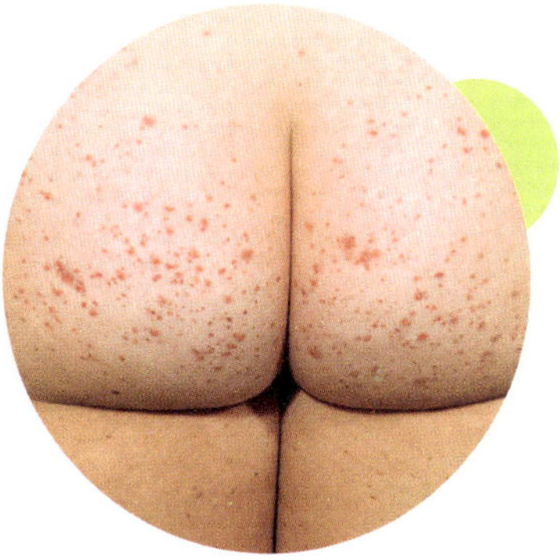

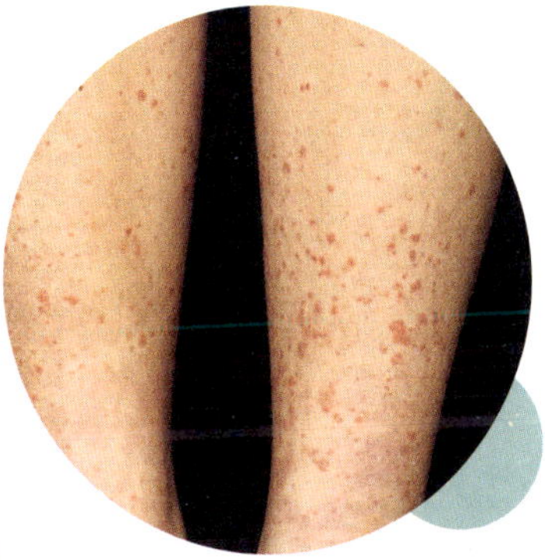

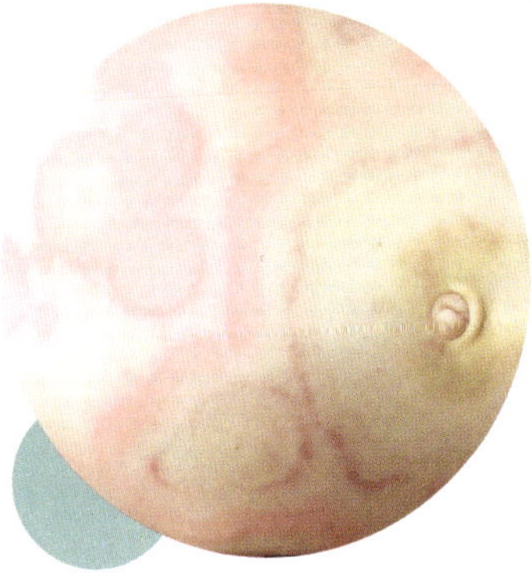

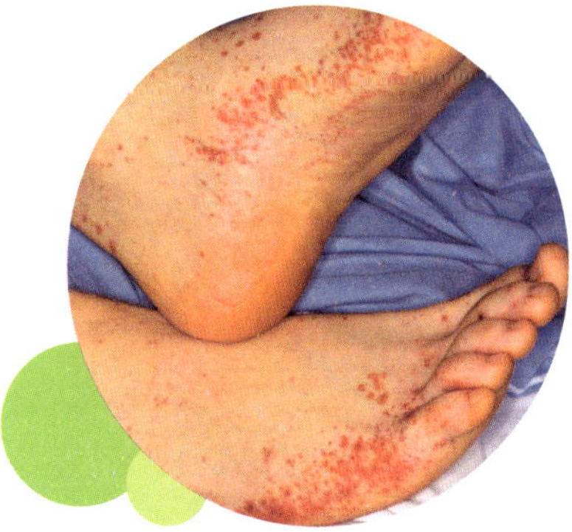

- **Joint pain and swelling:** Joint pain and swelling are common in children with HSP, particularly in the knees and ankles. This can cause difficulty walking or discomfort with movement.
- **Abdominal pain:** Abdominal pain is another frequent symptom, often accompanied by nausea, vomiting and sometimes blood in the poo. This can be quite distressing for both the child and the parents.
- **Kidney problems:** Some children with HSP develop mild kidney complications, usually in the form of blood or protein in the urine. In most cases, this resolves on its own. In rare instances, more serious kidney disease can arise.

Diagnosing HSP: the detective work

If your child exhibits any of the symptoms mentioned above, especially the characteristic rash, it's important to consult your doctor promptly.

We'll conduct a thorough evaluation, considering:

- **Medical history:** We'll ask about recent illnesses, medications, and any family history of HSP or similar conditions.
- **A physical examination:** We'll carefully examine your child's skin, joints and abdomen for signs of inflammation and other symptoms.
- **Laboratory tests:** These may include urine tests to check for blood or protein, blood tests to assess inflammation and kidney function, and possibly a skin biopsy to confirm the diagnosis.

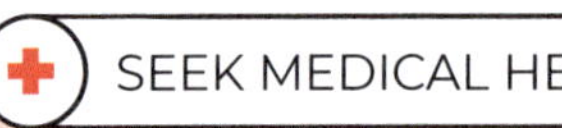

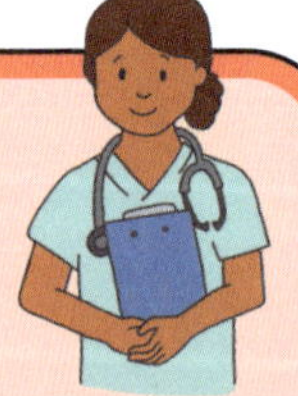

While most cases of HSP resolve without any lasting complications, it's important to seek immediate medical attention if your child experiences:

- severe abdominal pain that doesn't improve
- blood in the vomit or poo
- difficulty breathing or swallowing
- swelling of the face or tongue
- any other signs of severe illness.

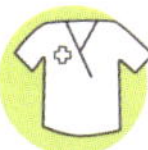

Treatment and management at home

Currently, there's no specific cure for HSP, but the focus of treatment is on managing the symptoms and monitoring for potential long-term complications.

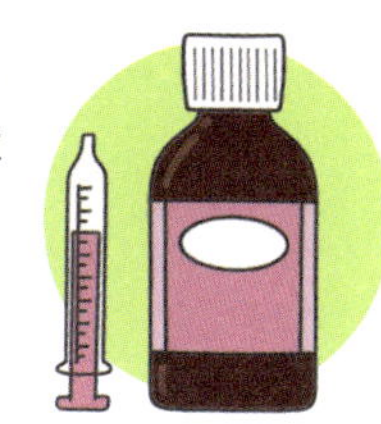

1. **Pain relief:** Over-the-counter pain relievers like paracetamol or ibuprofen can help relieve joint pain. Your doctor may prescribe stronger pain medications if needed.
2. **Rest:** Encourage your child to rest and stay hydrated to aid their body in healing.
3. **Monitoring:** Regular follow-up appointments with your child's doctor are essential to monitor kidney function, blood pressure and any other potential complications.
4. **Medications:** In some cases, if the symptoms are severe or if there's kidney involvement, your doctor may prescribe corticosteroids or other medications.

The road to recovery: what to expect

Most children recover from HSP within four to six weeks. However, the rash may come and go for several weeks or even months. Recurrences of HSP are possible but not common. With proper care and monitoring, your child can return to their normal activities and enjoy a healthy, active life.

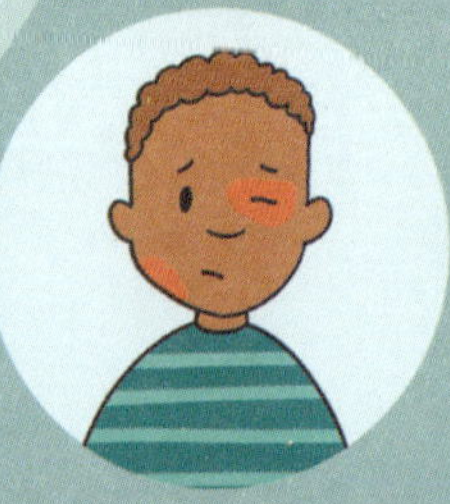

Skin infections

School sores (impetigo)

As a paediatrician, I see my fair share of itchy, crusty sores on kids. But there is one particular infection that parents should be aware of: school sores, also known as impetigo. This common and highly contagious bacterial skin infection needs antibiotics. While the lesions might look confronting, the good news is that impetigo is usually easy to treat and rarely causes serious complications; it almost never even leaves a scar.

SYMPTOMS: SMALL RED BUMPS OR BLISTERS THAT QUICKLY BURST, LEAVING BEHIND OOZING SORES

What are school sores?

Impetigo is a skin infection typically caused by *Staphylococcus aureus* or *Streptococcus pyogenes* (strep A, group A streptococcus) bacteria. These bacteria thrive in warm, humid conditions and can easily spread through direct contact with sores or contaminated objects. This is why impetigo is often called 'school sores' – it tends to spread quickly among children in close contact at childcare, kinder and school.

Who is most at risk of school sores?

While anyone can get impetigo, it's most common in children, particularly those between the ages of two and five. The term 'school sores' reflects the extremely contagious nature, as it spreads easily among preschool and school-aged children. Kids with eczema or other skin conditions that cause breaks in the skin are more susceptible.

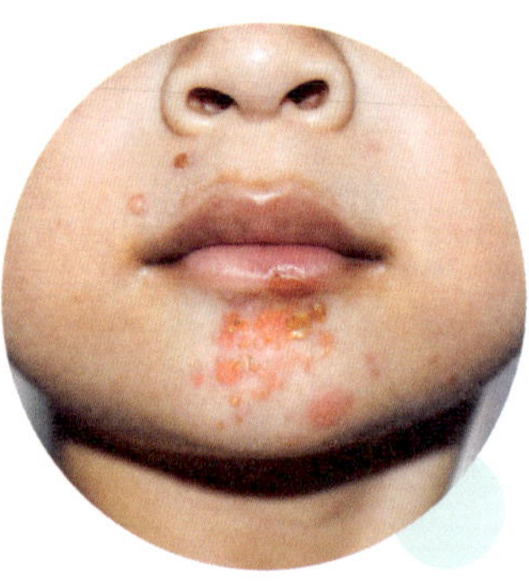

Recognising the signs

- Impetigo usually starts as small red bumps or blisters that quickly burst, leaving behind oozing sores.

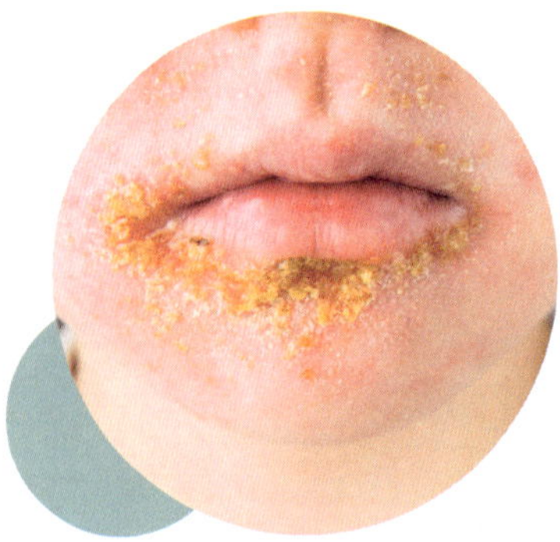

- These sores then crust over with a honey-coloured or yellowish-brown scab.
- The sores can be itchy and uncomfortable, but usually aren't painful unless they become infected or are scratched to the point of bleeding.

Where do school sores usually appear?

You'll most often find impetigo around the nose and mouth, but it can also affect other areas, like the arms, legs, bottom or genital area.

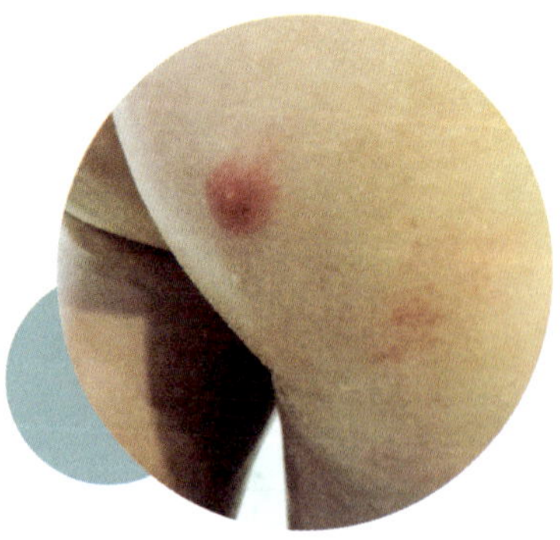

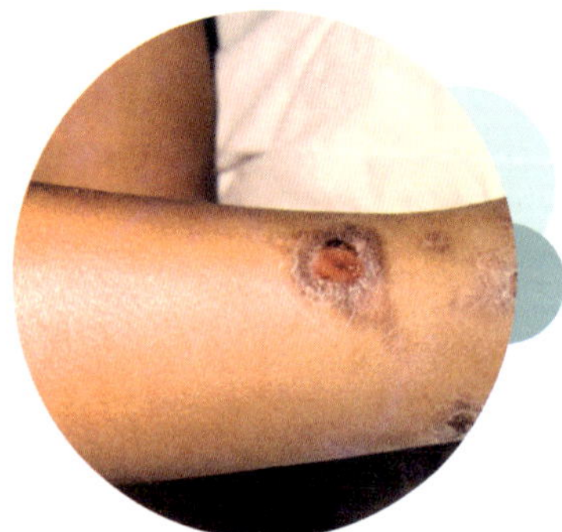

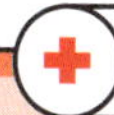

SEEK MEDICAL HELP

While most cases of impetigo are mild, contact your local doctor if:

- the sores worsen or don't improve after a few days of treatment
- your child develops a fever or other signs of illness
- the infection spreads to other parts of the body
- your child has a weakened immune system
- if you are concerned about potential abscess (a build-up of pus, a bit like a huge pimple) formation.

If your child gets frequent, recurrent sores, especially if they are associated with abscess formation and it's been found to be caused by methicillin-resistant *Staphylococcus aureus* (MRSA) then there may be a role for attempted 'decolonisation' or reduction of bacterial burden. You could discuss this with your doctor.

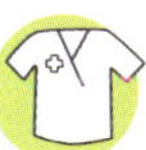

Treatment and management at home

Treatment for impetigo depends on the severity and extent of the infection.

1. **Mild cases:** Applying an over-the-counter antibiotic ointment to the sores for five to seven days is often enough. This will fix the vast majority of impetigo cases.
2. **More extensive cases:** Your doctor may prescribe an oral antibiotic to help clear the infection.
3. **Soaking and cleaning:** Gently soak the crusts with warm water and soap to help soften and remove them. This can make the antibiotic ointment more effective, as it reaches infected sore without being blocked by the scab.
4. **Bleach bath:** A daily 10-minute bleach bath may help to reduce the number of bacteria on your child's skin and reduce the risk of the impetigo spreading.

See pg. 168

Protecting others: containment is key!

Impetigo is highly contagious, so it's important to take precautions.

1. **Handwashing:** Encourage your child to practise good hand hygiene, especially after touching the sores.
2. **Isolate personal items:** Don't share towels, washcloths or other personal items with your child while they have impetigo.
3. **Keep your child's nails short:** Long nails can harbour bacteria and make it easier to spread the infection through scratching.
4. **Stay home:** Keep your child home from school or childcare until the sores are dry and no longer oozing, or for twenty-four hours after starting antibiotic treatment.

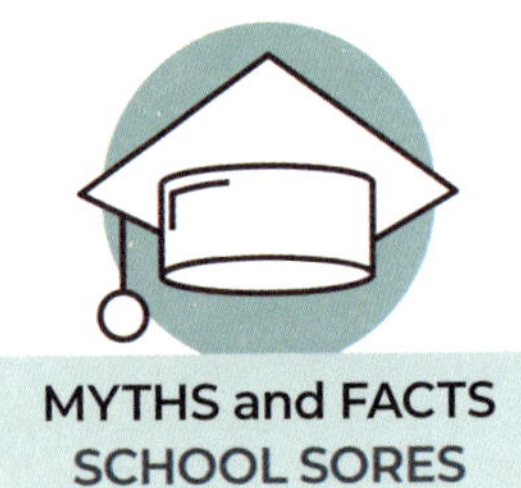

MYTHS and FACTS
SCHOOL SORES

Myth: Impetigo is caused by poor hygiene.

Fact: While good hygiene is important, anyone can get impetigo. It's caused by bacteria that can be present on healthy skin and spread through contact.

Myth: Impetigo is always serious.

Fact: Most cases are mild and easily treatable. However, in rare cases, impetigo can lead to more serious complications if left untreated.

Childcare or school exclusion

It is best for your child to remain home until appropriate treatment has started. When they return, any sores on exposed skin need to be covered with a watertight dressing.

Remember: Early treatment can help prevent the spread of impetigo and speed up healing. With proper care, your child will be back to their usual self in no time. If you have any concerns, don't hesitate to reach out to your local doctor or paediatrician. We're always here to help!

Skin infections

Molluscum

One of the more common referrals I see as a paediatrician is children with small, pearly bumps on their skin. These bumps are very easy to recognise, and they're caused by a common viral infection called molluscum contagiosum. While the name might sound a bit intimidating, it's usually a harmless condition that resolves on its own in time. Let's delve into what molluscum is, how it spreads, and what you can do as a parent.

SYMPTOMS: SMALL, ROUND, FLESH-COLOURED BUMPS

What is molluscum contagiosum?

Molluscum contagiosum is a skin infection caused by a bug from the poxvirus family. It's most common in children between the ages of one and ten, but can affect people of all ages, especially those with weakened immune systems.

How does molluscum spread?

The virus spreads through direct skin-to-skin contact with someone who has the bumps. It can also be transmitted through contact with contaminated objects, like towels, clothing or toys.

Molluscum LOVES to live in small, warm puddles of water, so it's extremely common to get outbreaks in summer, when children have swimming lessons or sit on the edge of a pool, where molluscum thrives in the surrounding puddles. Shared baths or swimming pools are probably the most common routes of transmission.

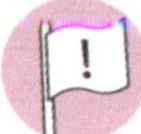

Recognising the signs

Molluscum bumps are small, round and flesh-coloured. They often have a pearly appearance and a tiny dimple or indentation in the centre. The bumps can appear anywhere on the body, but they're most common on the face, trunk, arms and legs.

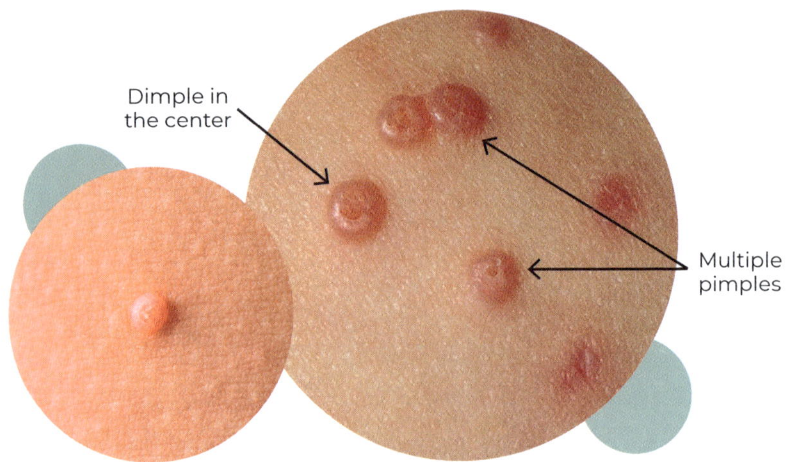

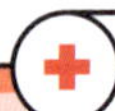

SEEK MEDICAL HELP

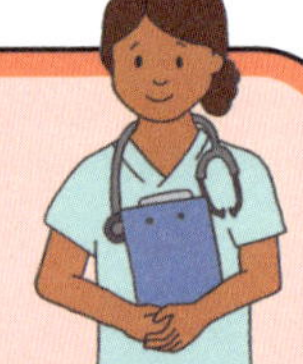

While most cases of molluscum are harmless, you should consult your doctor if:

1. **Your child has a weakened immune system:** Children with compromised immune systems may have more severe or persistent cases.
2. **The bumps are widespread or causing discomfort:** Treatment may be recommended in these cases.
3. **The bumps become infected:** Look for signs of redness, swelling, warmth or pus.
4. **You're worried:** If you're not sure whether your child has molluscum or not.

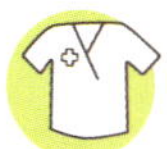 Treatment and management at home

The funny thing about molluscum is that it's probably the world's most unimpressive virus. It is so slow-moving and causes so few problems that the body takes months and months to even notice that it's there. When it eventually does find it, the process of beating it is equally slow, because it doesn't cause much of a threat. So I tell parents not to expect complete clearance for more than twelve months!

While molluscum usually clears up on its own, there are treatment options available if the bumps are bothersome, widespread, unsightly or are irritating pre-existing eczema or causing discomfort.

These include:

1. **Topical treatments:** Your doctor may prescribe creams or liquids that can help remove the bumps. Some treatments cause a small local reaction – to try to wake up the body's immune system and hasten its clearance.
2. **Physical removal:** Procedures like curettage (scraping), cryotherapy (freezing) and laser therapy can be used to remove the bumps.

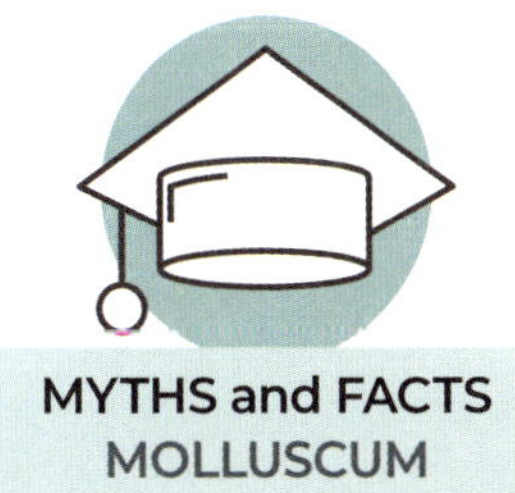

MYTHS and FACTS
MOLLUSCUM

Myth: Molluscum is sexually transmitted.

Fact: While molluscum can be transmitted through sexual contact in adults, it's most commonly spread through non-sexual contact.

Myth: Molluscum is a sign of poor hygiene.

Fact: Molluscum is caused by a virus, not by dirt or poor hygiene. Anyone can get it, regardless of how clean they are.

Myth: Molluscum needs to be treated immediately.

Fact: In most cases, molluscum resolves on its own without treatment within six to eighteen months.

Protecting others: reducing the spread

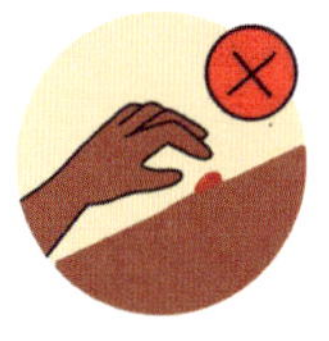

- Teach your child not to touch or pick at the bumps.
- Don't share towels, clothing or other personal items with people who have molluscum.
- Cover the bumps with a bandage if they are in areas that might be easily scratched or rubbed.
- Avoid siblings sharing baths or swimming pools if your child has open sores from molluscum. Cover affected areas if attending public swimming pools.

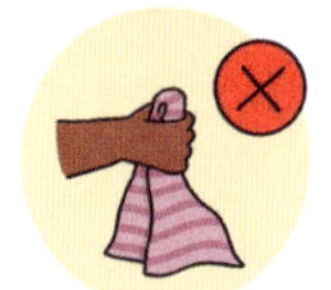

Childcare or school exclusion

There is no need to exclude a child with molluscum.

Remember: Molluscum contagiosum is a common and usually harmless childhood skin condition. While it can be frustrating, it's important to be patient and provide support to your child as their body fights off the virus. If you have any concerns, don't hesitate to talk to your local doctor.

Skin infections

Scabies

While scabies may sound like some medieval malady, it is well and truly alive and seen relatively often in paediatrics.

If your child is itching like crazy, especially at night, it might not just be dry skin or a mosquito bite. It might be a skin infestation caused by tiny mites, which we call scabies. While it can be a nuisance – and terribly itchy for the affected child – it's often easily treatable. Let's dive into the details so you can recognise, manage and get rid of the itch.

SYMPTOMS: INTENSE ITCHING, A RASH OF SMALL, RED BUMPS

What is scabies?

Scabies is caused by microscopic mites called *Sarcoptes scabiei*. These mites burrow into the top layer of skin, lay eggs and cause an intensely itchy rash. Scabies is highly contagious and can spread quickly through close personal contact, especially between family members and among children in childcare or school settings. It also spreads easily via infected bedding, clothing or towels.

Recognising the signs

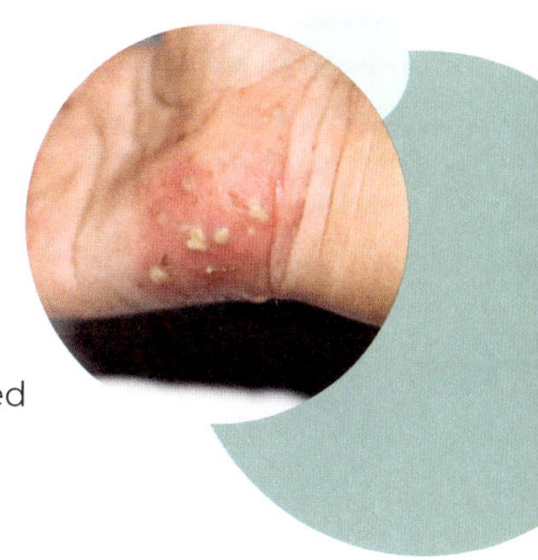

- **Intense itching:** This is the hallmark symptom of scabies, and it often worsens at night.
- **Rash:** The rash appears as small, red bumps, often with thin, raised lines (burrows) where the mites have tunnelled under the skin.

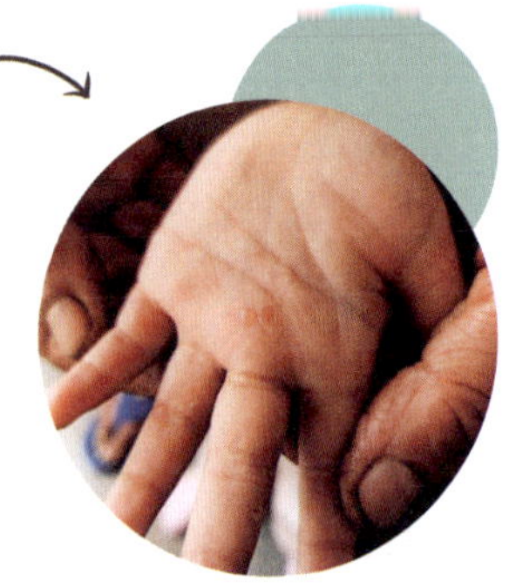

- **Location:** Scabies commonly affects the hands (especially between the fingers), wrists, elbows, armpits, waistline and genitals. In infants and young children, it can also appear on the head, neck, palms and soles of the feet.

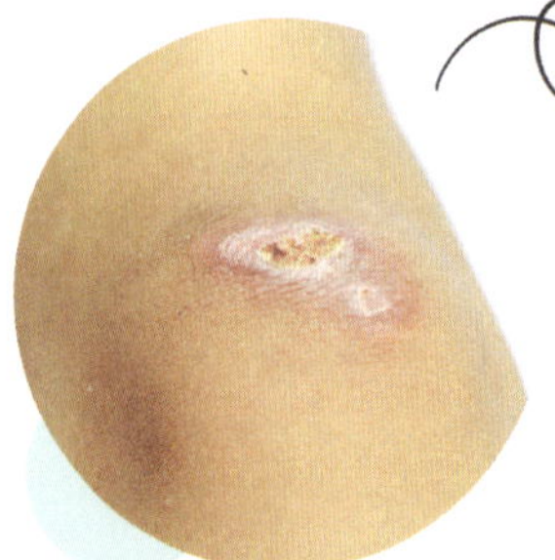

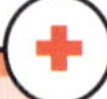

- **Secondary infections from scratching excessively:** Scratching can lead to bacterial infections, causing the sores to become crusty or filled with pus.

SEEK MEDICAL HELP

If your child has an itchy rash, especially if it's accompanied by the signs mentioned above, it's important to see your doctor for diagnosis. Early treatment can help prevent complications and stop the spread of the infestation.

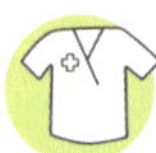

Treatment and management at home

If you suspect your child has scabies, it's important to see your doctor for diagnosis and treatment. Here's what you can expect:

- **Prescription medication:** Your doctor will usually prescribe a topical cream or lotion containing medications that kill both the mites and their eggs.
- **Entire household treatment:** Everyone in the household – and other close contacts – need to be treated at the same time, even if they don't have symptoms.
- **Wash everything:** All bedding, clothing and towels used by the infected person should be washed in hot water and dried on high heat to kill any remaining mites.

Protecting others: containment is crucial

- **Avoid close contact:** Encourage your child to avoid close contact with others who have scabies.
- **Wash hands frequently:** Good hand hygiene can help reduce the risk of transmission.
- **Don't share:** Avoid sharing personal items like towels, bedding or clothing with people who have scabies.

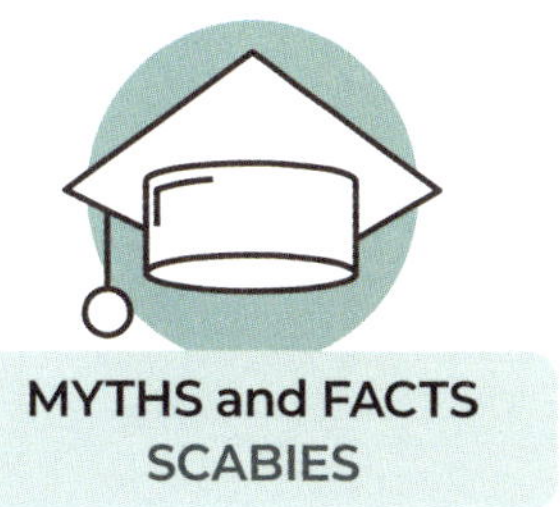

Myth: Scabies only affects people living in poverty.

Fact: Scabies can affect people of all socioeconomic backgrounds and living conditions. Outbreaks do occur in hotels and hostels, though, through inadequately cleaned bedding.

Myth: Scabies is a sign of poor hygiene.

Fact: Anyone can get scabies, regardless of their cleanliness. It's simply an infestation of mites, not a reflection of personal hygiene.

Myth: You can get scabies from pets.

Fact: While animals can have their own type of mite infestation, it's not the same as human scabies and can't be transmitted to humans.

Childcare or school exclusion

Your child should remain home until the day after starting appropriate treatment.

Remember: Scabies is a common and treatable condition. With the right treatment and preventive measures, you can help your child get relief from the itching and get back to their normal activities in no time.

Eczema

One of the most common – and underestimated – conditions of childhood is eczema, or atopic dermatitis. As a paediatrician, I know how distressing this condition can be for both children and parents; it's one of the most common causes of unsettled behaviour and poor sleep in babies! The good news is that we have a lot of tools and strategies to help manage eczema and improve your child's quality of life.

SYMPTOMS: DRY, RED, SCALY PATCHES OF SKIN; INTENSE ITCHING; SMALL RAISED BUMPS OR BLISTERS

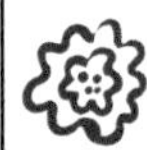

What is eczema?

Eczema is a chronic inflammatory skin condition that's incredibly common in kids. It's best thought of as a condition of extreme skin dryness. It's characterised by dry, itchy and red patches of skin that can flare up from time to time. While it's not contagious, eczema can be very uncomfortable, frustratingly itchy and even painful for little ones.

Understanding the causes of eczema

Eczema sometimes acts like a puzzle, with multiple pieces contributing to its development:

1. **Genetics:** If you or your partner has a history of eczema, allergies or asthma, your child is more likely to develop eczema as well. Think of it as a genetic predisposition.

2. **Skin-barrier dysfunction:** Eczema-prone skin has a weakened outer layer, making it difficult to retain moisture and protect against irritants. This allows allergens and bugs to enter the skin more easily, triggering inflammation and sometimes infection.

3. **Immune system imbalance:** The immune system plays a crucial role in eczema. In children with eczema, the immune system overreacts to triggers, leading to the characteristic inflammation and itching.

4. **Environmental triggers:** While not the root cause, various triggers can worsen eczema symptoms. These include certain soaps, foods, detergents, medicines, fabrics, allergens like dust mites or pollen, dry air, heat, sweat and even stress.

Recognising the signs and symptoms

Eczema can look different in each child and can vary depending on their age and the severity of the condition. Eczema typically appears on the face, scalp, torso, elbows, knees in babies, and in the creases of elbows, wrists, neck, knees, ankles in older children and adults.

Common signs and symptoms include:

- dry, red, scaly patches of skin (the skin feels almost like sandpaper)
- intense itching
- small raised bumps or blisters (which may ooze or crust over)
- thickened, leathery skin in areas that have been scratched repeatedly.

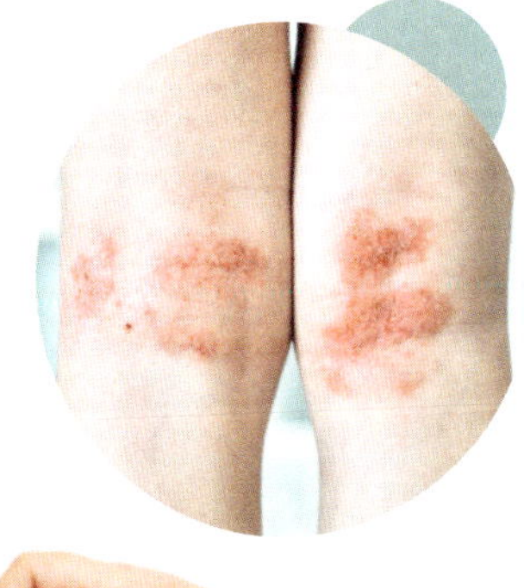

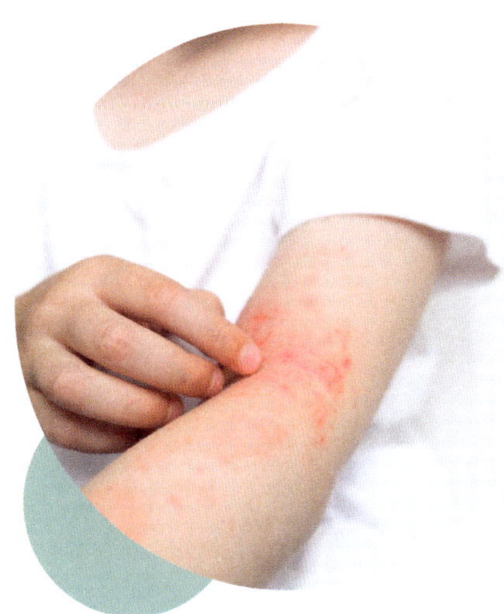

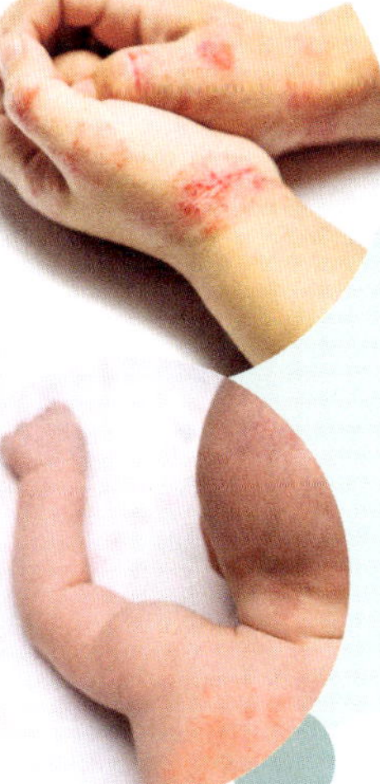

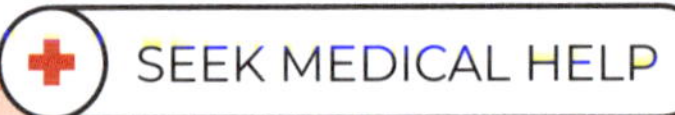

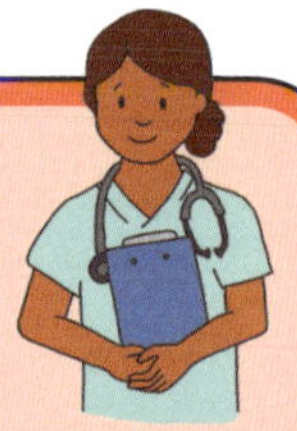

While many cases of eczema can be managed at home, it's important to consult your local doctor, paediatrician or dermatologist if:

- your child's eczema is severe, widespread or not responding to home treatment
- the itching is so intense that it interferes with your child's sleep or daily activities
- you notice signs of infection, such as redness, swelling, heat or pus
- your child's eczema is affecting their emotional wellbeing or self-esteem.

MYTHS and FACTS ECZEMA

Myth: Eczema is just dry skin.

Fact: While dry skin is a symptom, eczema is a complex inflammatory condition and the physical discomfort should not be underestimated.

Myth: Eczema is caused by poor hygiene.

Fact: Eczema is not related to cleanliness. In fact, excessive washing or using harsh soaps can strip the skin's natural oils, making eczema worse, especially in young babies.

Myth: Eczema is contagious.

Fact: Eczema cannot be caught from another person.

A note on heat

Given that eczema is essentially extreme dryness, the number-one enemy of eczema is heat. To prevent overheating, try removing a single layer (clothing or blanket) from your child, while also ensuring they never get too cold. Clothing made of natural fibres and breathable fabric is preferable.

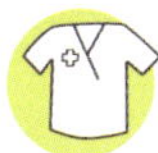

Treatment and management at home

Eczema is a chronic condition, meaning it doesn't have a cure. But we have a wide range of effective strategies to manage it and reduce flare-ups. Most children will grow out of eczema – some entirely, others mostly – with only the occasional flare triggered by a stressor.

1. **Moisturisers:** The cornerstone of eczema management! Apply a thick, fragrance-free moisturiser several times a day to hydrate and protect the skin.
2. **Topical (applied directly to skin) steroids:** These anti-inflammatory medications can help reduce redness, swelling and itching during flare-ups. They come in different strengths and can carry side effects if used for too long, so always use them under the guidance of your doctor.
3. **Other topical medications:** Depending on the severity of the eczema, your doctor may prescribe other topical medications, which provide an alternative to steroid creams and ointments.
4. **Oral medications:** In severe cases, oral medications like antihistamines, steroids or immunosuppressants may be considered.
5. **Wet dressing therapy:** This soothing technique involves applying moisturiser and wet bandages to the affected areas. It's particularly helpful for severe flare-ups. While messy and uncomfortable, it's like a magic treatment for eczema exacerbations!
6. **Trigger avoidance:** Identifying and avoiding triggers that worsen your child's eczema is crucial for long-term management.
7. **Bleach baths:** Diluted bleach baths can help reduce bacteria on the skin, which can reduce infection risk and improve eczema.

Remember: You're not alone in this journey! With a proactive approach, proper treatment and a good understanding of your child's triggers, you can help them manage eczema and enjoy a happier, healthier childhood.

How to give a bleach bath

What you'll need for a bleach bath:

1. Household bleach, 4.2 per cent sodium hypochlorite (e.g. White King);
   - do not use fragranced (e.g. lemon- or lavender-scented) bleach
2. Measuring cup
3. Standard-sized bucket (10 L)
4. Waterproof tape or a marker

Step 1:

Fill the bath with tap water to the desired level using the 10 L bucket. Count the number of buckets you use.

Step 2:

Mark your bath with waterproof tape or a marker. (This is so you don't need to use the bucket next time.)

Step 3:

Add 12 ml of bleach for every bucket (10 L) of water. This gives a final bleach concentration of 0.005 per cent.

Step 4:

Let your child soak in the bath for ten minutes.

Step 5:

Wash your child's head and face with the bath water. But do not submerge their head in the water. Avoid direct contact too close to the eyes.

Step 6:

Wipe away any crusting or weeping at infected areas while your child is in the bath. Use a soft, disposable towel (e.g. a Chux-type cloth) and throw it away afterwards.

TIPS:

- Do not rinse your child's skin after the bath.
- Use old or white towels to avoid possible bleaching of coloured towels.
- Repeat the bleach baths as often as recommended by your child's doctor or nurse.
- For eczema management, moisturise the child immediately after the bath.

Possible side effects:

- Household bleach can sometimes cause a stinging or burning sensation on the skin, but this recipe is for a very diluted bath so it's less likely.
- If your child does have stinging or irritation in the diluted bleach bath, rinse them off with plain water. Discuss this with your child's doctor or nurse before giving them another bleach bath.

Remember: This may sound excessive, and most parents are horrified when I recommend bleach baths, but they are widely (and safely) used in paediatrics to treat skin infections. The key is to get the dilution correct – the final bleach concentration is lower than in a swimming pool, so if you're happy to jump in a pool, there's no need to worry about a bleach bath.

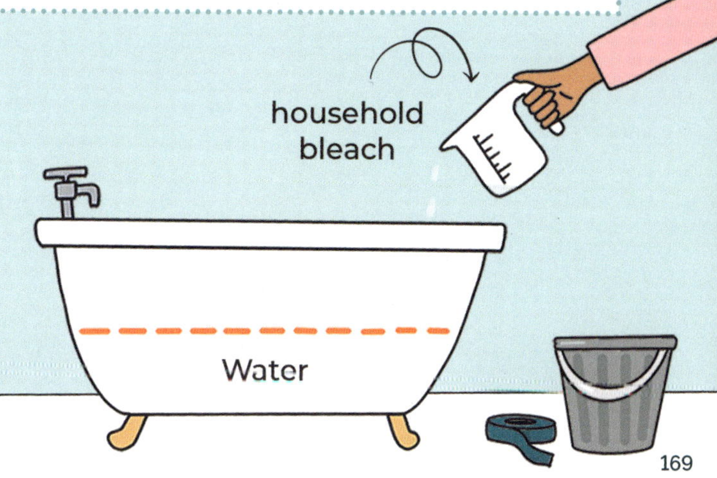

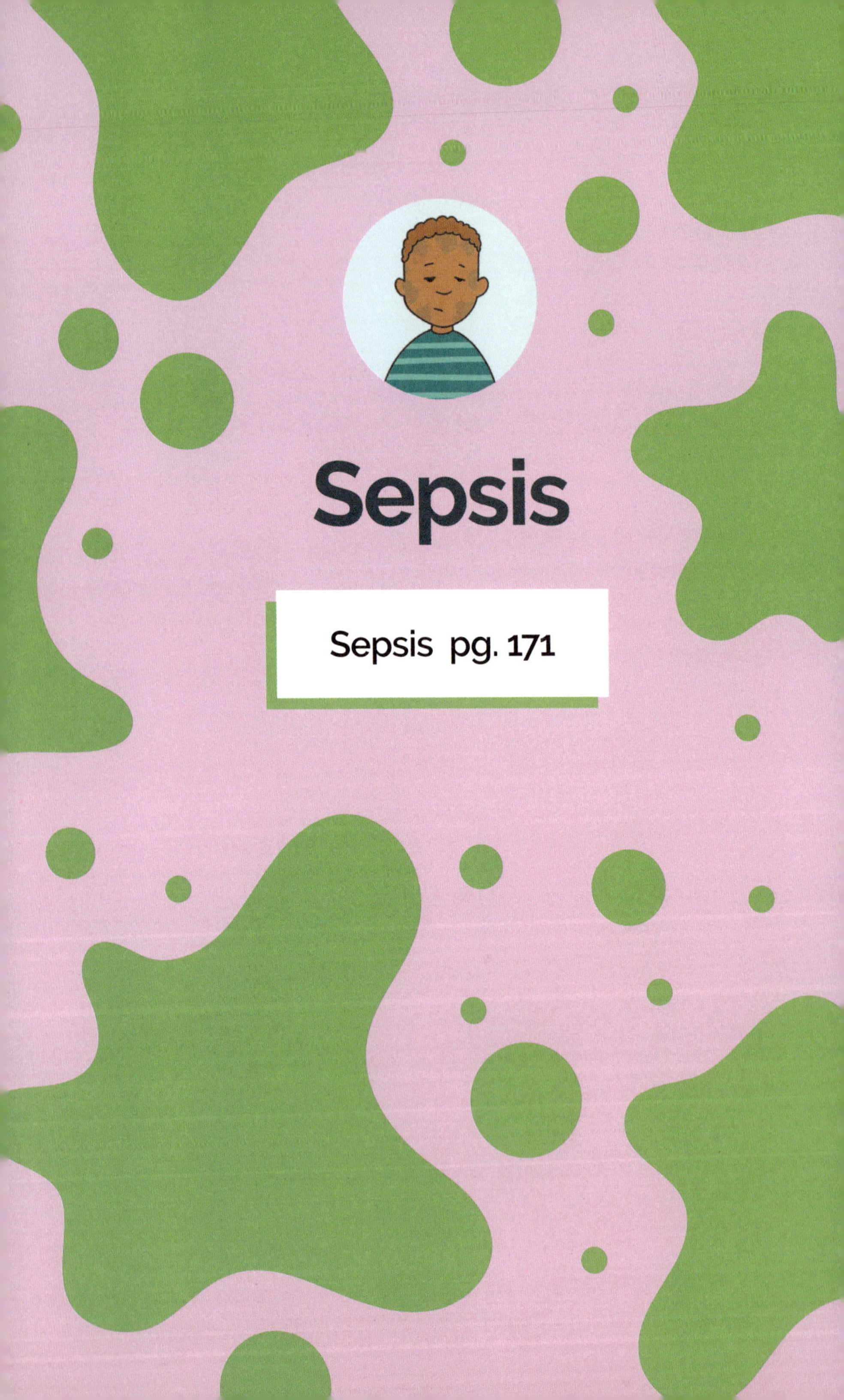

Sepsis

Sepsis

Sepsis

One of the most critical conditions I watch for in children is sepsis. It might not be as familiar as the common cold or an ear infection, but it's incredibly important to understand, as early recognition and treatment are crucial. While the thought of sepsis can be scary, clear information and guidance will help you protect your child.

SYMPTOMS: FEVER; FAST HEART RATE AND BREATHING; LETHARGY OR EXTREME SLEEPINESS; POOR FEEDING OR FEWER WET NAPPIES; COOL, CLAMMY SKIN; CHANGES IN MENTAL STATE

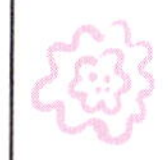

What is sepsis?

Sepsis is an uncommon life-threatening condition that occurs when the body's response to an infection goes into overdrive. Instead of just fighting the infection, the immune system starts attacking the body's own tissues and organs, in an overreaction to the original threat. This can lead to organ failure and even death if not treated promptly; time is of the essence.

How does sepsis happen?

Sepsis can develop from any type of infection, whether it's bacterial, viral or fungal. Common original sources of infection include the lungs, urinary tract, skin and blood. In young children, sepsis often starts with a seemingly mild infection that quickly escalates. It's not common, but it is very serious.

Who is most at risk of sepsis?

While sepsis can affect anyone, certain groups of children are at higher risk, including:

- newborns and infants under three months of age
- children with weakened immune systems
- children with chronic medical conditions
- children recovering from surgery or injury.

Recognising the symptoms

Early recognition of sepsis is vital, but the symptoms can be tricky, especially in young children, as they often overlap with other common illnesses. Here are some red flags to watch for:

- **Fever:** This is a common sign of infection, but with sepsis it can be very high or accompanied by chills or shakes (rigors).
- **Skin changes:** Rashes can occur (petechiae and purpura) from the infection causing the sepsis (such as meningococcal, see page 144), though they can also occur due to disruptions to the body's clotting ability when really unwell. Other skin changes like mottling may result from dehydration.
- **Fast heart rate and breathing:** These are signs that the body is working hard to fight the infection.
- **Lethargy or extreme sleepiness:** Your child may be unusually tired or difficult to wake up.
- **Poor feeding or fewer wet nappies:** Infants may have trouble feeding or produce less urine.
- **Cool, clammy skin:** This can be a sign of poor circulation.
- **Changes in mental state:** Your child may be confused, irritable or less responsive than usual.
- **Nausea, vomiting and diarrhoea:** Severe sepsis can mimic a gastro-like illness, however this would never be the only sign but part of a constellation of other concerning symptoms and signs.

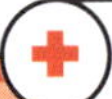

SEEK URGENT MEDICAL HELP

If you notice any of these signs in your child, especially in combination, it's crucial you seek medical attention immediately. Time is of the essence when it comes to sepsis. Don't hesitate to call for emergency services.

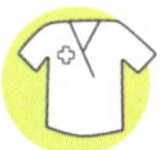

Treatment: a race against time

Sepsis requires urgent medical care. In the hospital, your child will be assessed and may receive:

- **Intravenous fluids:** To maintain blood pressure and organ function.
- **Antibiotics:** To fight the infection.
- **Other medications:** To manage complications, like low blood pressure.
- **Oxygen:** If your child has difficulty breathing.
- **Close monitoring:** To track their vital signs and ensure their condition is improving.

Prevention

While not all cases of sepsis can be prevented, there are steps you can take to reduce your child's risk:

- **Vaccinations:** Ensure your child is up to date on all recommended vaccines, as these can protect against some of the infections that can lead to sepsis.
- **Prompt treatment of infections:** If your child shows signs of an infection, seek medical attention promptly. Early treatment can often prevent complications.
- **Good hygiene:** Teach your child to wash their hands frequently and avoid close contact with sick people.
- **Optimise health:** Maximise your child's sleep quantity and quality, and encourage a clean and balanced diet.

Remember: While sepsis is a serious condition, early recognition and treatment significantly improve outcomes. As a paediatrician, I encourage you to trust your instincts and seek medical attention if you have any concerns about your child's health.

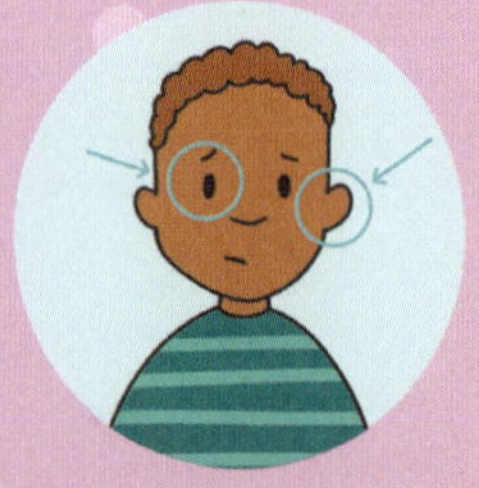

Eyes and ears

Ear infections and grommets

If your child is tugging at their ears, has a fever or seems fussier than usual, they might have an ear infection. Ear infections are one of the most common reasons general practitioners see young children in practice. While most ear infections resolve on their own, sometimes they can become recurring or persistent, leading to the possible need for a procedure called tympanostomy tube insertion, better known as grommets. Let's explore this condition and what you can do as a parent if you suspect it's affecting your child.

SYMPTOMS: EAR PAIN, FEVER, IRRITABILITY AND DIFFICULTY SLEEPING, FLUID DRAINING FROM THE EAR, HEARING DIFFICULTIES

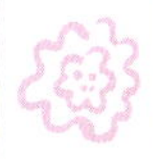

What are ear infections?

Ear infections (known as acute suppurative otitis media, or ASOM) are infections of the middle ear, the air-filled space behind the eardrum. It's often caused by upper respiratory viruses or bacteria that enter the middle ear through the Eustachian tube, a narrow passage that connects the middle ear with the back of the throat. When this tube becomes blocked or inflamed, fluid can build up behind the eardrum, creating an ideal environment for germs to grow.

Why are children more prone to ear infections?

Young children are more susceptible to ear infections because of their developing immune systems and the anatomy of their Eustachian tubes. Their tubes are shorter, narrower and more horizontal than those of adults, making it easier for fluid to become trapped and for germs to enter. It's also harder for children to clear their Eustachian tubes.

Recognising the symptoms

- **Ear pain:** This is the most common symptom, especially in older children. Younger children may tug at their ears or become increasingly fussy.
- **Fever:** Often accompanies an ear infection, especially in babies and toddlers.
- **Irritability and difficulty sleeping:** The discomfort from ear pain can disrupt children's sleep and make them irritable.
- **Fluid draining from the ear:** You may notice a clear, white or yellow discharge from the ear, which suggests a perforated ear drum.
- **Hearing difficulties:** A build-up of fluid in the middle ear can temporarily impair hearing.

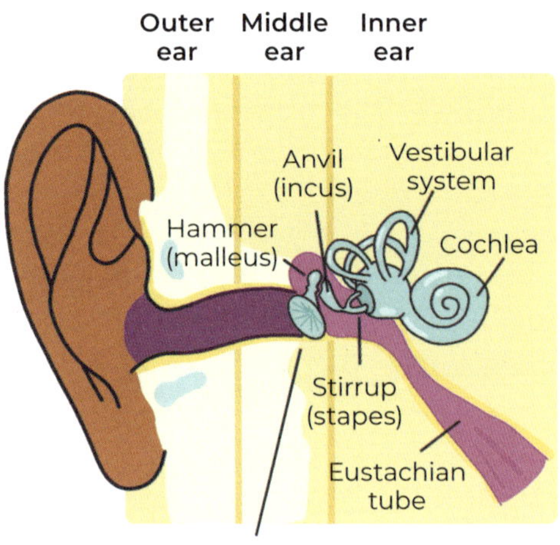

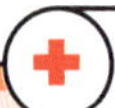

SEEK MEDICAL HELP

If you suspect your child has an ear infection, it's important to see your doctor for diagnosis and treatment. They can examine the ear using an otoscope (special torch) and recommend the best course of action. Most ear infections are caused by viruses and resolve on their own within a few days, without antibiotics. However, some may require antibiotics and pain relief, especially if the symptoms are severe or persistent.

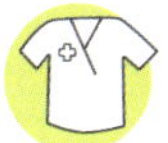

Treatment and management at home

Here are some things you can do to help your child feel better and manage their symptoms:

- **Hydration:** Encourage your child to drink plenty of fluids, such as water, breastmilk, formula, oral rehydration solution or clear broth. This helps keep them hydrated and can loosen mucus.
- **Saline:** Saline drops or spray can help loosen mucus and soothe irritated nasal passages. Then use a nasal aspirator for young children.
- **Humidifier:** A cool-mist humidifier can moisten the air and make breathing easier.
- **Pain and fever relief:** If your child has a fever or is uncomfortable, over-the-counter medications like paracetamol or ibuprofen can be helpful. Always follow the recommended dosage for your child's age and weight.
- **Rest:** Make sure your child gets plenty of rest, as their body needs energy to fight off the virus.
- **Elevate the head of the bed:** Slightly elevating the head of your child's bed can help with drainage and make breathing easier at night. This is not advised for babies. Always ensure you are following safe-sleep tips for younger children.

What are grommets?

In some cases, children experience recurring or persistent ear infections, or fluid build-up behind the eardrum that doesn't clear on its own. We call this 'glue ear'. In these situations, your doctor may recommend the insertion of grommets, also known as tympanostomy tubes.

Grommets are tiny tubes that are surgically placed into the eardrum. They look like mini-doughnuts and create a small opening that allows air to enter the middle ear and fluid to drain out. This can help reduce the frequency of painful ear infections and improve hearing.

When are grommets recommended?

Your doctor may recommend grommets if your child:

- has had multiple ear infections within a short period (for example, three or more in six months)
- has persistent fluid in the middle ear that hasn't cleared after several months
- experiences hearing loss due to fluid build-up, confirmed by audiology (hearing) and tympanometry (pressure) testing.

What to expect: grommet insertion and aftercare

Grommet insertion is a relatively simple procedure performed under general anaesthesia. The tubes usually fall out on their own within six to eighteen months, and the eardrum typically heals without scarring. After the procedure, your doctor may recommend ear drops to prevent infection and advise against getting water in the ears while swimming or bathing.

> A very common scenario that occurs in my rooms is the finding that children referred for language delay actually have recurring ear infections and glue ear. One of the first things we do is have an audiologist assess the child's hearing and eardrum movement. Remember, we're not talking about complete hearing loss – it's a loss of frequency, so the child hears things as if they are underwater. It's not nothing, but it's not clear, and you need clear hearing at all frequencies to achieve language development.

Childcare or school exclusion

There is no need for exclusion.

> ✱ **Remember:** Your doctor is there to guide you through any concerns you have about your child's ear health. If you suspect an ear infection or have questions about grommets, don't hesitate to reach out to your doctor.

Eyes and ears

Conjunctivitis

Conjunctivitis, also known as pink eye, is a common eye condition affecting children of all ages.

SYMPTOMS: PINK OR RED EYES; WATERY, STICKY OR THICK DISCHARGE; ITCHING OR BURNING SENSATION; GRITTY FEELING IN THE EYES; SENSITIVITY TO LIGHT; CRUSTING AROUND THE EYELIDS

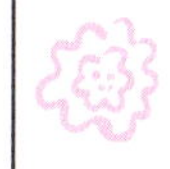

What is conjunctivitis?

Conjunctivitis is simply an inflammation or infection of the conjunctiva, which is the transparent membrane that covers the white part of the eye and lines the eyelids. Think of it like a little blanket for your eye. When this blanket gets irritated, it can cause a range of symptoms.

What are the types of conjunctivitis?

There are three main types of conjunctivitis:

1. **Viral conjunctivitis:** This is the most common type, often caused by the same viruses responsible for the common cold. It's incredibly contagious but usually clears up on its own within a week or two. Your child might have watery eyes, redness and maybe some mild irritation.

2. **Bacterial conjunctivitis:** Caused by bacteria, this type can be treated with antibiotic eye drops or ointment prescribed by your doctor. It's contagious but less common than viral conjunctivitis. Along with eye redness, your child might have thicker, stickier discharge, especially after sleep.

3. **Allergic conjunctivitis:** If your child has allergies, their eyes might react to pollen, dust mites, pet dander or other allergens. This isn't contagious, but it can cause intense itching, watery eyes and sometimes swelling of the eyelids.

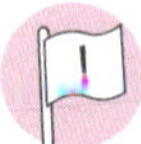

Recognising the symptoms

- Pink or red eyes
- Watery, sticky or thick discharge
- Itching or burning sensation
- Gritty feeling in the eyes
- Sensitivity to light
- Crusting around the eyelids, especially in the morning.

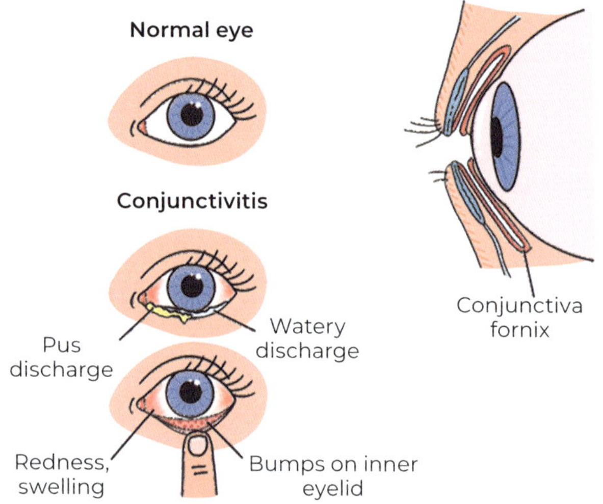

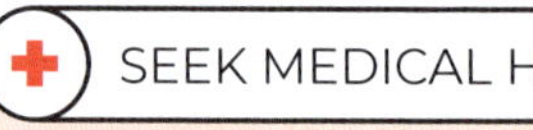

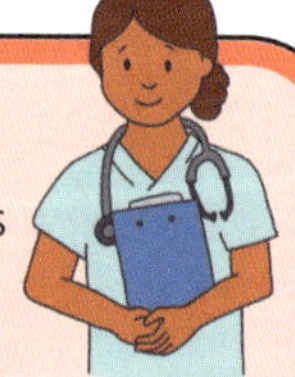

In most cases, conjunctivitis is mild and resolves quickly. However, seek immediate medical attention if your child:

- has severe eye pain
- experiences changes in vision
- has redness or swelling that worsens rapidly
- is less than one month old and shows any eye symptoms
- only one eye is really red, especially if associated with pain, swelling or weeping.

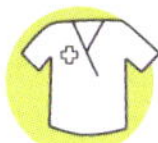

Treatment and management at home

1. **See your doctor:** They'll determine the type of conjunctivitis and recommend the appropriate treatment.
2. **Practise good hygiene:** Frequent handwashing is crucial. Avoid sharing towels, washcloths and pillows. Don't touch the infected eye.
3. **Follow treatment instructions:** If your doctor prescribes medication, use it as directed.
4. **Manage allergies:** If it's allergy-related, try to identify and avoid triggers. Over-the-counter antihistamine eye drops may help.

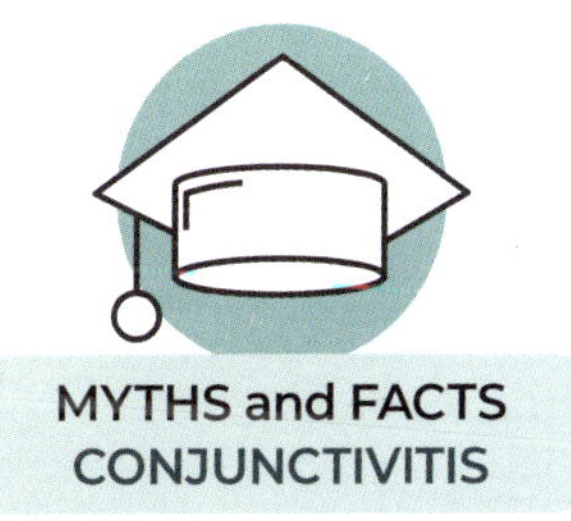

Myth: Breastmilk can cure conjunctivitis.

Fact: While breast milk undoubtedly has many benefits, there's no scientific evidence to support this. If your newborn has sticky eyes, they might have blocked tear ducts – which we'll cover next.

Myth: All conjunctivitis is contagious.

Fact: Only viral and bacterial conjunctivitis are contagious.

Myth: You need antibiotics if you have conjunctivitis.

Fact: Antibiotics are only necessary for bacterial conjunctivitis.

Childcare or school exclusion

Children should remain home until the discharge from their eyes has stopped.

Keep your child home: If it's viral or bacterial conjunctivitis, they should stay home from school or childcare until the discharge is gone to prevent spreading it to others.

Blocked tear ducts

Blocked tear ducts – nasolacrimal ducts – are a very common issue in infants. It can be a little worrying to see your baby's eyes constantly watering or crusting over, but rest assured, it's usually a harmless condition that resolves on its own.

SYMPTOMS: WATERY EYES, STICKY OR CRUSTY DISCHARGE, REDNESS OR SWELLING

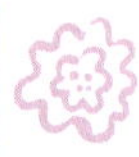

What is a blocked tear duct?

Our eyes produce tears to keep them moist and clean. These tears drain into the nose through tiny channels called tear ducts, which are located in the inner corner of the eyelids. In some babies, these ducts may not be fully open at birth, leading to a blockage.

Why do tear ducts get blocked?

In most cases, it's simply a matter of the tear duct not opening fully before birth. The tissue at the end of the duct can be narrow or covered by a thin membrane. It's like a tiny plumbing issue that usually corrects itself as your baby grows.

Who does it affect?

Blocked tear ducts are most common in newborns and infants under six months old. However, it can occur in older babies as well. We generally don't surgically treat blocked tear ducts until twelve to eighteen months of age.

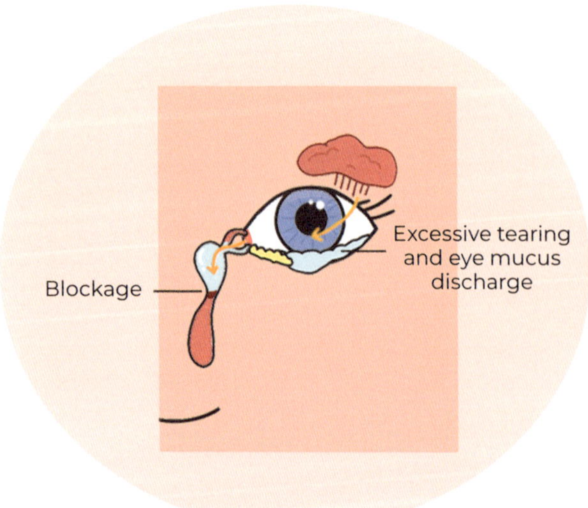

Recognising the symptoms

- **Watery eyes:** One or both eyes may appear constantly teary, even without crying.
- **Sticky or crusty discharge:** You might notice a yellowish-white discharge around the eyes, especially after sleep.
- **Redness or swelling:** The skin around the eye may be slightly red or puffy.
- **Recurrent eye infections (conjunctivitis):** While less common, blocked tear ducts can sometimes lead to infections.

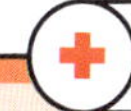

SEEK MEDICAL HELP

While most blocked tear ducts resolve spontaneously, consult your local doctor if:

- your baby is over twelve months old and still has symptoms
- the eye becomes increasingly red, swollen or painful
- the discharge turns green or yellow, suggesting an infection
- your baby has a fever or seems unwell.

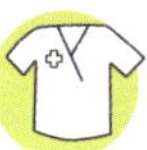

Treatment and management at home

1. **Tear duct massage:** You can gently massage the area over the tear duct several times a day. This can help open the blockage.
2. **Warm compresses:** Applying a warm, damp cloth to the affected eye can help loosen any discharge and soothe irritation.
3. **Wiping the eye from the inside to the outside:** Use a cotton pad or cotton-wool ball soaked in warm tap water (you do not need to use saline or sterile eye wipes from the pharmacy) and wipe gently from the inside of the eye to the outside. Once used, dispose of the cotton-wool ball, without reusing.

4. **Antibiotic eye drops (if needed):** If your baby develops an eye infection, your doctor might prescribe antibiotic drops. These are extremely overprescribed, so please only use them if there are signs of infection.

5. **Surgery:** Rarely, an ophthalmologist (a specialist eye surgeon) will pass a small probe through the tear duct while the patient is under anaesthetic to open the duct manually.

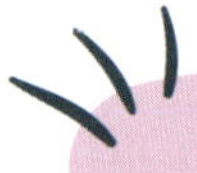

The vast majority of babies with a blocked tear duct will respond perfectly to warm tap water and a cotton-wool ball.

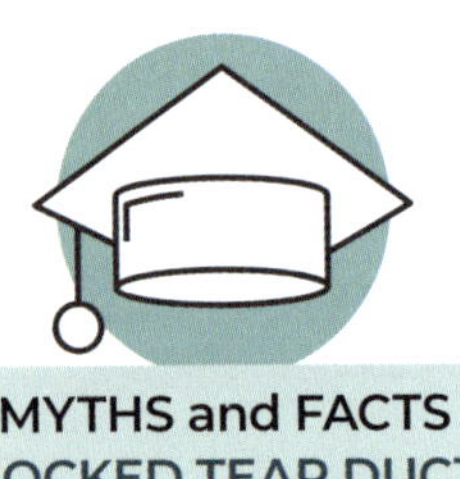

MYTHS and FACTS
BLOCKED TEAR DUCTS

Myth: Blocked tear ducts always require surgery.

Fact: Most cases resolve on their own within the first year of life. Surgery is rarely necessary.

Myth: Blocked tear ducts are caused by something the mother did during pregnancy.

Fact: This is not true. It's a structural issue, unrelated to anything the mother did.

Myth: Breastmilk will fix blocked tear ducts.

Fact: Breastmilk belongs in the mouth! There is no need and no benefit in squirting breastmilk into your baby's eyes.

Childcare or school exclusion

There is no need for exclusion.

Remember: Patience is key! With time and simple measures like massage and warm compresses, most blocked tear ducts clear up on their own.

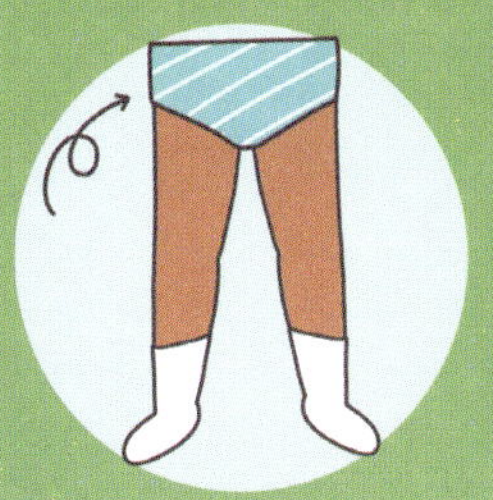

Under pants

UTI: urinary tract infection pg. 186

Pinworms pg. 189

UTI: urinary tract infection

Urinary tract infections are a common concern in my practice. While they can be a bit alarming for parents, the good news is that with prompt recognition and treatment, most children recover quickly and without complications. Let's delve into what UTIs are, how to spot them and what you can do as a parent to help your child.

SYMPTOMS: PAIN OR BURNING DURING URINATION, FREQUENT URINATION, ABDOMINAL PAIN, FOUL-SMELLING URINE, FEVER

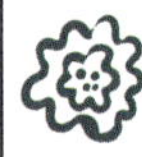

What is a UTI?

A UTI is an infection that occurs anywhere in the urinary tract – the system that produces, stores and eliminates urine. This includes the kidneys, ureters (the tubes that carry urine from the kidneys to the bladder), bladder and urethra (the tube that carries urine out of the body) in both boys and girls. Most UTIs in children affect the bladder and urethra, known as lower UTIs.

Why do children get UTIs?

UTIs happen when bacteria enter the urinary tract and multiply. Young children, especially girls, are more prone to UTIs due to their shorter urethras, which make it easier for bacteria from the outside world to reach the bladder. Other factors that can increase the risk include:

1. **Toilet training:** Holding urine for too long can allow bacteria to multiply.
2. **Constipation:** Stool build-up can put pressure on the bladder and make it harder to empty completely.
3. **Bubble baths:** Soaps and bubble baths can irritate the urethra and make it easier for bacteria to enter.

4. **Structural abnormalities:** In some cases, anatomical issues in the urinary tract can increase the risk of UTIs. Young babies will often undergo an ultrasound scan of their renal system, to ensure the structures are normal.
5. **Poor hygiene practices:** This is especially important in girls. Please always teach children to wipe front to back.

Recognising the signs and symptoms

UTIs can be tricky to spot in young children, as their symptoms may not be specific. Young babies may only exhibit feeding disturbance or lethargy, without the more common symptoms of fever, discernible pain or foul-smelling urine.

Here are some signs to watch for in older babies and children:

1. **Pain or burning during urination:** Your child may cry or complain of discomfort while urinating.
2. **Frequent urination:** They may need to go to the toilet more often than usual, even if they only pass small amounts of urine.
3. **Urgency:** They may have a sudden, strong urge to urinate.
4. **Wetting accidents:** Children who are toilet-trained may start having accidents.
5. **Abdominal pain:** They may complain of pain in the lower abdomen or back.
6. **Foul-smelling urine:** The urine may have a strong, unpleasant odour.
7. **Fever:** UTIs can sometimes cause a fever, especially in younger children.

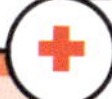

SEEK MEDICAL HELP

If your child shows any of these signs, it's important to see your doctor for diagnosis and treatment. A simple urine test – performed on the spot – can usually confirm the presence of a UTI.

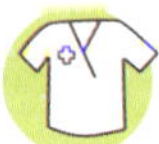

Treating UTIs: antibiotics to the rescue

UTIs are treated with antibiotics, which usually clear the infection within a few days. It's essential to complete the entire course of antibiotics as prescribed by your doctor, even if your child starts feeling better sooner. This helps ensure that the infection is completely eradicated, reduces the risk of recurrence and minimises antibiotic resistance.

Prevention

While not all UTIs can be prevented, there are steps you can take to reduce your child's risk:

1. **Encourage good hygiene:** Teach girls to wipe from front to back after using the toilet and to wash their hands thoroughly.
2. **Promote regular urination:** Encourage your child to empty their bladder completely and regularly, rather than holding it for long periods. Tactical wees are great for preventing UTIs. (Also to avoid having to go to a public toilet after you leave the house!)

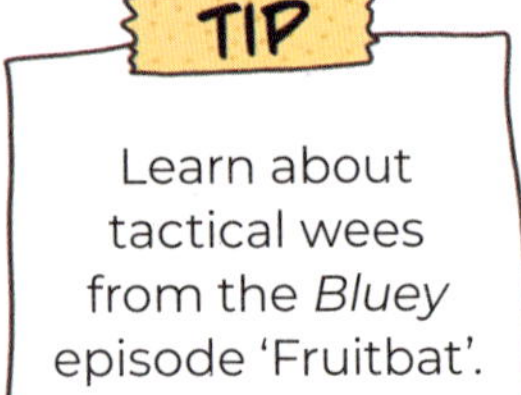

3. **Stay hydrated:** Make sure your child drinks plenty of fluids throughout the day.
4. **Limit bubble baths:** Stick to plain water or mild, non-irritating soaps.
5. **Address constipation:** If your child is constipated, work with your doctor to manage it effectively.
6. **Cotton underwear:** Underwear made of synthetic materials increases the risk of getting an UTI.

Childcare or school exclusion

There is no need for exclusion.

Remember: UTIs are common in children, but with prompt diagnosis and treatment, they can be easily managed. Your paediatrician will always answer your questions and guide you through any concerns you may have about your child's urinary health.

Under pants

Pinworms

As a paediatrician, I often encounter kids who are itching around their bottoms, especially at night. Still, I didn't realise just how distressing this can be until I witnessed it in my own children.

While there can be several culprits, one common cause is pinworms, tiny parasites that can create an annoying and sometimes embarrassing problem. But rest assured, pinworms are very common, especially among young children, and they're easily treatable. Let's delve into the details so you can understand, manage and banish these unwelcome guests.

SYMPTOMS: ITCHING AROUND THE BOTTOM, RESTLESSNESS AND IRRITABILITY, TROUBLE SLEEPING, VAGINAL IRRITATION, ABDOMINAL PAIN

What are pinworms?

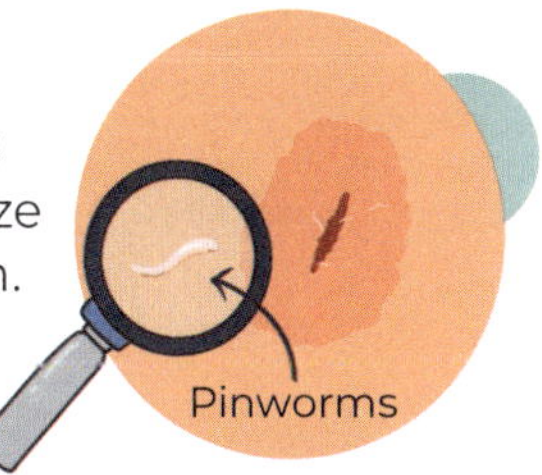

Pinworms are small, white, thread-like worms that infest the intestines. They're about the size of a staple – sometimes as small as an eyelash. If your child has an infection, you might see the pinworms around your child's bottom, especially at night, when the female pinworms come out to lay eggs. One female will lay more than 15,000 eggs over a two-week period! These eggs are tiny and invisible to the naked eye, but they're the main reason infections are so contagious.

How do pinworms spread?

Pinworm eggs can be found on contaminated surfaces like toys, bedding, toilet seats and even under fingernails. When someone touches these eggs and then puts their fingers in their mouth, they swallow the eggs, which then hatch and grow into adult pinworms in the intestines. The cycle continues when the female pinworms lay eggs around the anus, causing itching and leading to further contamination. The treatment requires destroying the pinworms *and* their eggs, to prevent further life cycles.

Recognising the signs and symptoms

While itching around the bottom, especially at night, is the most common symptom, other signs of pinworms can include:

1. **Restlessness and irritability:** The itching can disrupt sleep and make children irritable.
2. **Trouble sleeping:** Frequent waking due to itching is common.
3. **Vaginal irritation:** Pinworms can sometimes migrate to the vagina, causing itching and irritation. The pain and distress is very real and should not be dismissed.
4. **Abdominal pain:** This is less common but can occur.

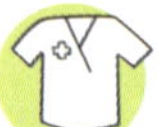

Treatment and management at home

A two-pronged approach: If you suspect your child has pinworms, see your doctor for diagnosis. Treatment usually involves two steps:

1. **Medication:** Your doctor will recommend an anti-parasitic medication to kill the pinworms; most are available without a prescription. This medication is usually a single dose, but a second dose is often given two weeks later to ensure all the worms are gone. Everyone in your household needs to take the medicine, even if they are asymptomatic.
2. **Hygiene measures:** To prevent reinfection, it's crucial to clean and disinfect your child's surroundings. Wash all bedding, towels and clothing in hot water and dry on high heat. Clean toilets, toys and frequently touched surfaces regularly. Vacuum to remove any residual eggs and clean all house surfaces, especially door handles. Always discourage children from eating food that has touched the floor and try to minimise thumb-sucking or hands entering the mouth.

Prevention

While it can be difficult to completely prevent pinworm infections, especially in childcare or school settings, here are some things you can do:

1. **Handwashing:** Teach your child to wash their hands thoroughly with soap and water after using the toilet, before eating and after playing outdoors.
2. **Nail hygiene:** Keep your child's nails short and clean.
3. **Regularly change your child's underwear and pyjamas:** This can help reduce the number of eggs present.
4. **Avoid scratching:** Encourage your child not to scratch their bottom, as this can spread the eggs.

MYTHS and FACTS
PINWORMS

Myth: You can catch pinworms from pets.

Fact: Pinworms are specific to humans and can't be caught from animals.

Myth: Pinworms are an indication of poor hygiene.

Fact: Pinworms are not a sign of poor hygiene; they are common in all socioeconomic groups and can affect anyone. They're not a reflection of cleanliness.

Childcare or school exclusion

There is no need for exclusion.

Remember: Pinworms are a common and treatable childhood problem. By understanding how they spread and taking preventive measures, you can help your child stay itch-free and healthy.

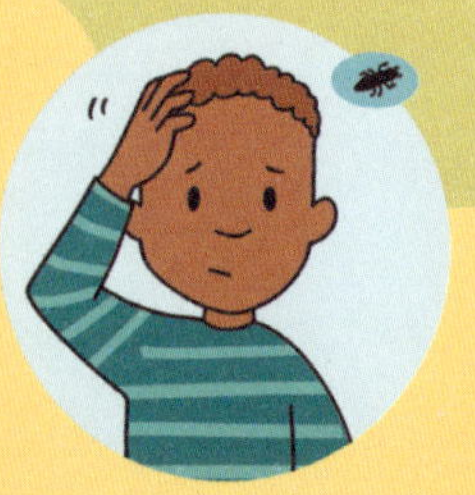

Other gross things

Oral thrush

Parents often come into my practice concerned about white patches in their baby's mouth. While the patches can be a bit alarming at first glance, they are most often just milk (breastmilk or formula) that collects in the tiny grooves and crevices of the tongue. They're harmless and can be wiped away, though they will return at the very next feed. Less frequently, these patches can be a sign of oral thrush (candidiasis), a usually harmless fungal infection. Let's explore what thrush is, why it happens in children, and how to manage it.

SYMPTOMS: WHITE PATCHES OR COATING ON THE TONGUE, INNER CHEEKS, GUMS OR ROOF OF THE MOUTH; REDNESS OR SORENESS; DIFFICULTY FEEDING OR FUSSINESS

What is oral thrush?

Oral thrush, also known as oral candidiasis, is caused by an overgrowth of a type of yeast called *Candida albicans*. This yeast is naturally present in small amounts in the mouth, but certain factors can trigger its excessive growth, leading to thrush.

Why do children get thrush?

Children, especially infants and toddlers, are more susceptible to thrush due to their developing immune systems.

Factors that can contribute to thrush in children include:

1. **Antibiotic use:** Antibiotics can disrupt the balance of bacteria and fungi in the mouth, allowing *Candida* to overgrow.
2. **Weak immune system:** Children with underlying medical conditions or those taking medications that suppress the immune system may be more prone to thrush.

3. **Inhaled corticosteroid use:** Inhaled steroids, often used for asthma or other respiratory conditions, can increase the risk.

4. **Poor oral hygiene:** While often not the primary cause, infrequent cleaning of bottles, pacifiers and toys can contribute to the growth of *Candida*.

Recognising the symptoms

Oral thrush typically presents as:

1. **White patches or coating on the tongue, inner cheeks, gums or roof of the mouth:** These patches may resemble cottage cheese and can be difficult to wipe off. They are usually quite plentiful, extensively covering the inner cheeks, tongue and palate.

2. **Redness or soreness:** The affected areas may be red, inflamed or tender.

3. **Difficulty feeding or fussiness:** Infants with thrush may be fussier than usual during feeding or refuse to eat due to discomfort. Breastfeeding mothers might experience nipple pain if the thrush infection passes from baby to mother.

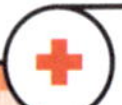

SEEK MEDICAL HELP

If you suspect your child has thrush, it's important to see your doctor for diagnosis and treatment. While thrush is usually mild, it's crucial to rule out other conditions that require different treatment. It is especially important for a young infant with (what seems to be) recurrent thrush to be seen by a doctor.

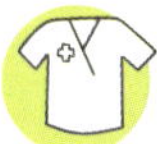 Treatment and management at home

Treatment for oral thrush usually involves:

1. **Antifungal medication:** Your doctor may prescribe an antifungal medication in the form of a liquid, gel or oral drops. This medication is typically applied directly to the affected areas several times a day, including to a breastfeeding mother's nipples.
2. **Good oral hygiene:** Cleaning your child's mouth regularly with a soft, damp cloth can help remove excess yeast and soothe discomfort.
3. **Cleaning or replacing pacifiers and bottle nipples:** If your child uses pacifiers or bottles, ensure they are thoroughly cleaned or replaced to prevent reinfection.
4. **Addressing underlying causes:** If your child has been taking antibiotics or using inhaled steroids, discuss with your doctor whether adjusting the medication or dosage could help.

Prevention

Some ways to help prevent oral thrush:

1. **Breastfeeding:** When possible, avoid prolonged periods of dampness by changing breast pads regularly.
2. **Proper bottle and nipple hygiene:** Clean bottles and bottle nipples thoroughly after each use.
3. **Limiting sugar intake:** Excessive sugar consumption can promote the growth of *Candida*.
4. **Appropriate use of antibiotics:** Broad-spectrum antibiotic use is a big risk for thrush. While these antibiotics have a role, it is okay to ask a doctor if the antibiotic is essential when it is prescribed.
5. **Rinsing of mouth after using inhaled corticosteroids:** It's often good to brush your child's teeth immediately after they use inhaled steroids to ensure adequate cleaning of the mouth.

Childcare or school exclusion

There is no need for exclusion.

Head lice

Head lice, often called nits, is formally known as *Pediculosis humanus capitis*. These tiny critters are a common nuisance in childhood, but with the right knowledge and approach, you can say goodbye to those itchy scalps and rest easy.

SYMPTOMS: ITCHY SCALP, SORES ON SCALP

What are head lice?

Head lice are tiny, wingless insects that live on the human scalp and feed on blood. They're not a sign of poor hygiene or uncleanliness; they can be found on anyone, regardless of how often they wash their hair.

Who gets head lice?

Head lice are most common in young children, especially those in childcare and primary school settings. They spread unbelievably easily through head-to-head contact during play or by sharing personal items like hats, combs, brushes or hair accessories.

Recognising the signs

- The most common symptom of head lice is an itchy scalp, especially behind the ears and at the nape of the neck.
- Not all kids get itchy, so spot checks during hair-brushing is good practice if they are at school or in a childcare setting. If there's an outbreak, do a quick check every day.
- You might also see sores on the scalp. Head lice don't cause sores themselves, but they can develop from scratching and may become infected.

Head-lice life cycle

The lice life cycle can be separated into three stages. Knowing about these stages can help you to identify what you're looking at when you do a 'nit check'.

Stage 1: eggs

While head lice are often referred to as 'nits', a nit is actually the tiny white or yellowish-brown egg, firmly attached (almost glued) to the hair shaft. These eggs are usually laid within 6 mm of the scalp. Once laid, they take between seven and thirteen days to hatch into a nymph.

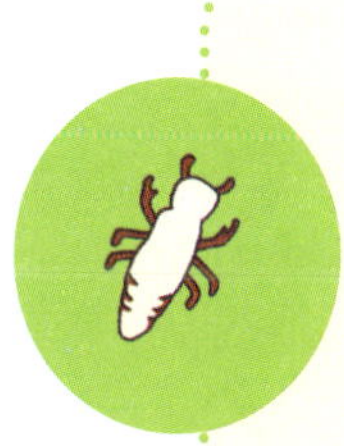

Stage 2: nymph

These are newly hatched baby lice. Nymphs look like adult lice but are about the size of a pinhead. It takes around seven to ten days for a nymph to mature into an adult louse capable of breeding.

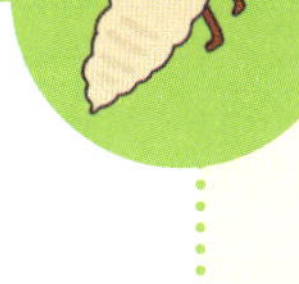

Stage 3: adult lice

Adult lice are tan to grey in colour. They have six legs ending in hook-like claws (perfect for holding on to hair). When fully grown, they are about the size of a sesame seed (up to 3 mm long). The female is slightly larger than the male and lives, on average, for thirty to forty days. Female lice produce an average of five eggs per day and can lay up to 150 eggs during their lifespan.

Head-lice life cycle

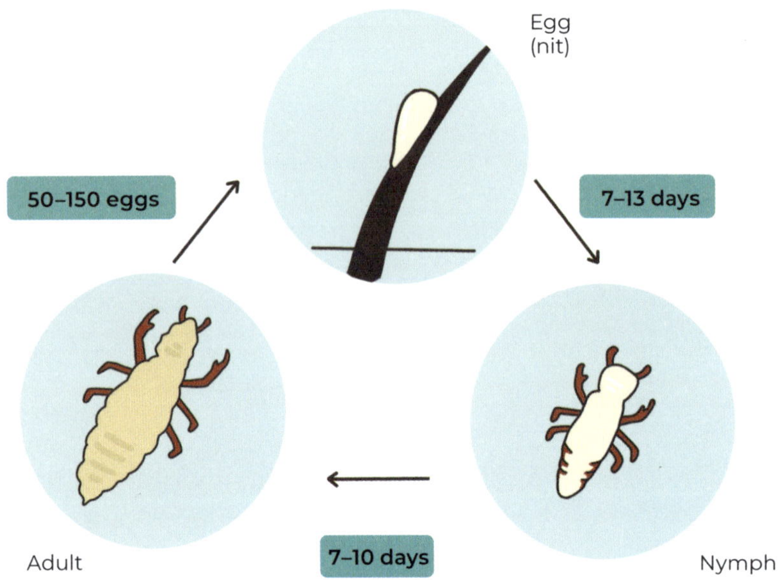

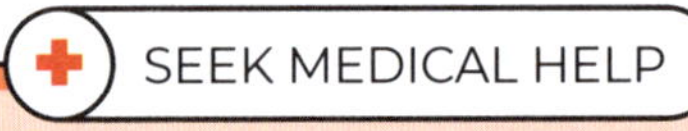

Most cases of head lice can be managed at home. However, you should consult your doctor if:

- your child is under two months old
- the infestation is severe or doesn't improve with over-the-counter treatments
- your child develops signs of a skin infection, such as redness, swelling or oozing sores.

How to check for nits

1. If there are live adult lice, they can be easy to spot – particularly in light-coloured hair. If there are only nits (eggs), it can be harder to identify, though somewhat easier to spot in darker-coloured hair.

   Spotting eggs: nits can be mistaken for dandruff but you can tell the difference because they are harder to remove – a bit of dandruff will 'flick off' whereas a nit will need to slide off the hair shaft with your nail or a fine-toothed nit comb.

2. If there's an outbreak at childcare or school, don't wait until your child is itchy (some kids never get itchy with lice). Check your child every night to stay on top of it – early detection will make treatment much simpler!

3. Good natural light is best for checking. If it's evening, use a torch or bright light.

4. Check the entire head, with a particular focus on the back of the neck and behind the ears.

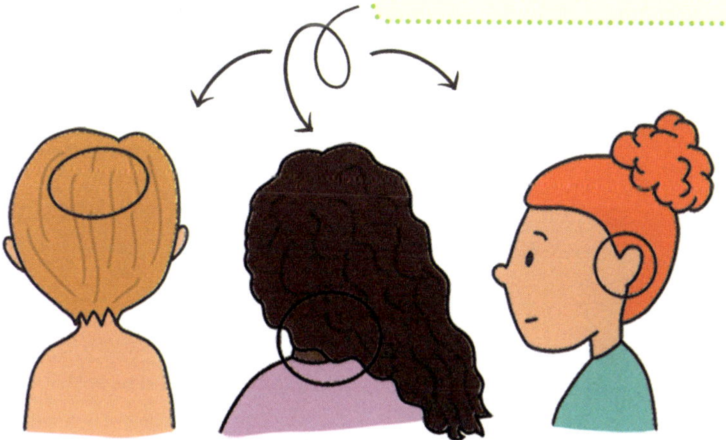

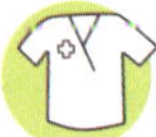

Treatment and management at home

Thankfully, head lice are treatable! I recommend a combination of both medical and mechanical removal.

Here's what you can do:

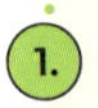

Medicated shampoos or lotions (medical removal): These over-the-counter treatments are designed to kill lice and nits. Follow the instructions carefully, and repeat the treatment as directed. Often you will be advised to do a second treatment a week after the first. The natural treatments from the pharmacy can be incredibly effective – oil-based products with spray-gun applicators are much easier to administer, particularly if you're treating a whole house. Often they will come with a comb and recommend mechanical removal as well.

Wet combing (mechanical removal): After using a medicated treatment, wet combing with a fine-toothed nit comb can help remove nits and dead lice. This process can be painstaking and time-consuming, but is very effective.

Step 1:

Massage a lot of conditioner through dry hair.

- Use a store-bought conditioner (get a cheap one as you'll be using a lot of it).
- The conditioner won't kill the lice but it will 'stun' them for about twenty minutes, making them easier to remove.

Step 2:

Give the hair a normal comb. This will get any knots out, so you're ready for the nit comb.

Step 3:

Get a bowl of hot water and a paper towel. Position the hot water carefully, to avoid any accidental burns.

Step 4:

You need to comb EVERY strand of hair. For long hair, it will be easier if you comb it in sections.

Step 5:

Rinse and wipe the comb.

- Each comb through, dip the comb in the hot water and wipe clean with the paper towel.
- Sometimes you may only get a nit or two – if it's a serious case, you will get many eggs and possibly some lice (hopefully they're all dead after the medicated treatment).

3. **Dry combing:** There are some great electric combs for dry combing. These are terrific for what I refer to as a 'quick sweep' – they'll catch any debris in the hair and let you know quickly if you've got a case of nits (they're also great for doing a quick sweep of your own hair if you're worried). I still recommend old-fashioned wet combing for the management of all confirmed cases of nits.

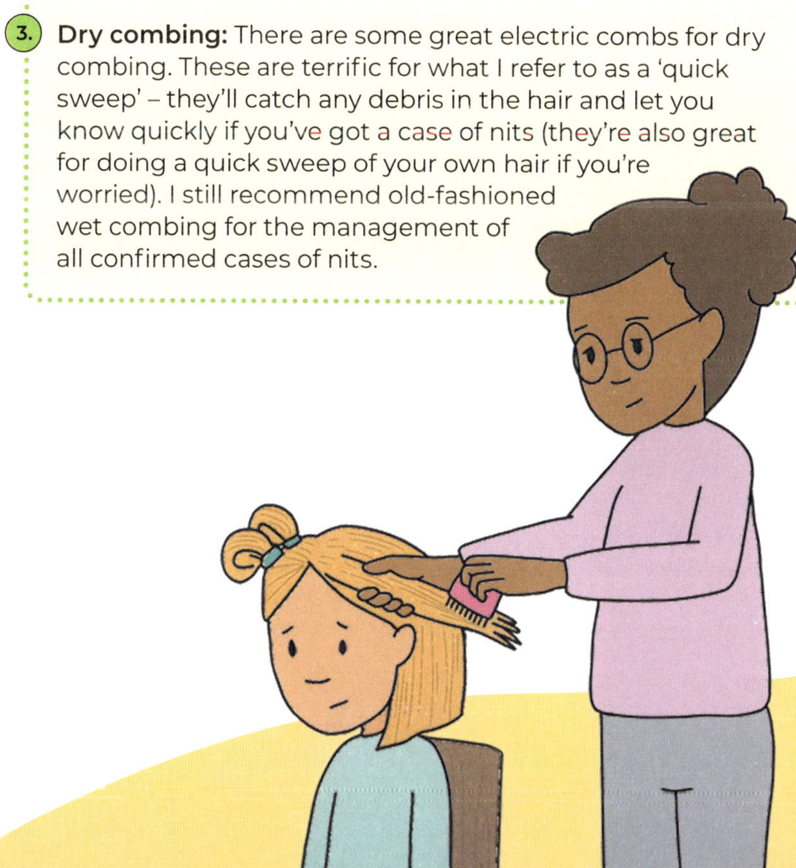

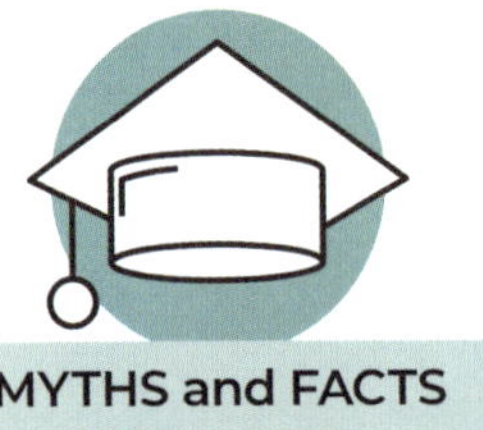

MYTHS and FACTS HEAD LICE

Myth: Head lice spread disease.

Fact: Head lice are not known to transmit any diseases.

Myth: Head lice can jump or fly.

Fact: Lice can only crawl; they cannot jump, fly or swim.

Myth: Head lice only affect people with long hair.

Fact: Head lice can affect anyone, regardless of hair length.

Myth: You need to hot wash every piece of material and bedding in your house on a high heat cycle if someone in the household has lice.

Fact: Head lice are only found on the human head or hair. To survive, they need to feed on blood several times a day. They quickly dehydrate and die if removed from the head, in about twenty-four to forty-eight hours. Head lice do not live on furniture, bedding, carpet or anywhere else in the environment. I recommend hot-washing pillow cases, towels, hats and hair accessories that have been used since the outbreak, but you don't need to go overboard; enough time away from a scalp will disable them.

Myth: If you have an itchy head, you have head lice.

Fact: Just reading this section will give you an itchy head – it can be very psychosomatic! Most of the time when you're searching for nits you'll realise a lot of your family have dry scalps which can cause itchiness too. This may be a sign of eczema or seborrheic dermatitis. If you're not sure, discuss with your doctor.

Prevention

1. **Keep long hair tied up and in plaits or braids:** This reduces the possibility of a new louse getting back in during an outbreak. You can use hairspray to slick the hair back. My tip is to use a small amount of store-bought conditioner to keep hair slightly greasy and damp when styling – it will stop wispy pieces from flying out and make it easier to comb. It'll look a little greasy but it's way better than nits!

2. **Avoid sharing personal items:** Discourage your child from sharing combs, brushes, hats and other hair accessories.

3. **Hygiene:** Wash pillow cases, towels and clothing in hot water and dry on high heat.

Childcare or school exclusion

There is no need for exclusion so long as effective treatment commences before the next school day.

✱ **Remember:** Head lice are a common nuisance, but they're not a health hazard. With patience, persistence and the right approach, you can get rid of them and keep them from coming back. If you have any concerns or questions, don't hesitate to talk to your doctor.

(Is it just me, or are you scratching your scalp now too?)

Ringworm (tinea)

The first – and most important thing – to say about ringworm is that this fungal infection is not caused by worms. It's called ringworm because the actual skin marking looks like a tiny worm. Let's delve into what ringworm is, how it spreads, and what you can do to help your child.

SYMPTOMS: RING-SHAPED RASH, ITCHING, SCALY SKIN, HAIR LOSS

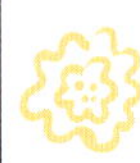

What is ringworm?

Ringworm – otherwise known as tinea – has different names depending on where it occurs in the body. It also has different appearances, depending on location. It is a fungal infection caused by dermatophytes; these fungi thrive in warm, moist environments and can infect the skin, scalp or nails.

Ringworm is highly contagious and can spread through direct skin-to-skin contact with an infected person or animal, or through contact with contaminated objects or surfaces.

There are five main variations of ringworm:

1. **Tinea pedis:** Also known as athlete's foot, this looks like dry, cracked skin between the toes and is incredibly itchy.

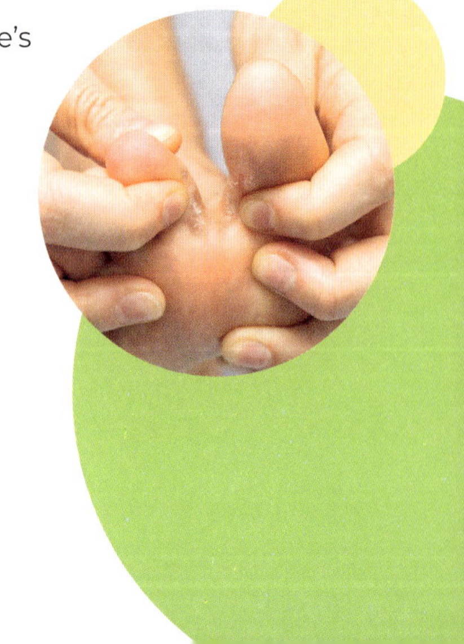

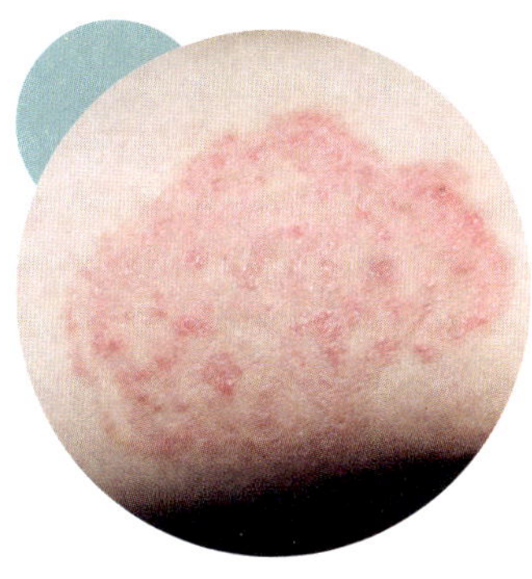

2. **Tinea corporis:** This can affect the skin anywhere in the body but is most commonly found on the trunk, arms and legs.

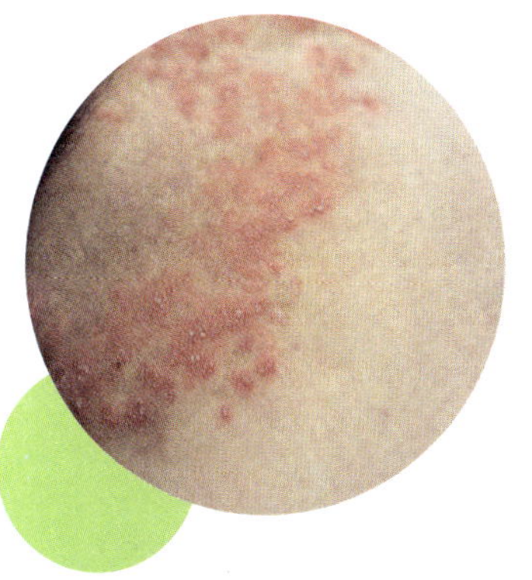

3. **Tinea cruris:** This appears in the groin, thus is often called jock itch, and begins as ring-shaped scaly rashes. It starts flat but slowly becomes raised and the inside of the ring becomes clear, so it looks like a shallow doughnut.

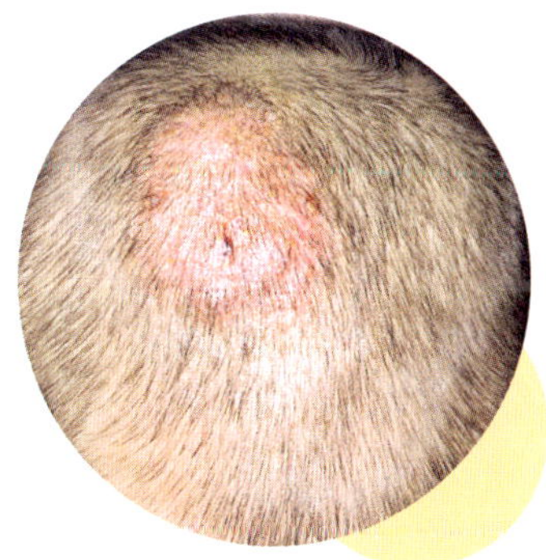

4. **Tinea capitis:** This appears on the scalp. You'll see a small pimple that slowly enlarges, with a surrounding area of hair loss and dry skin.

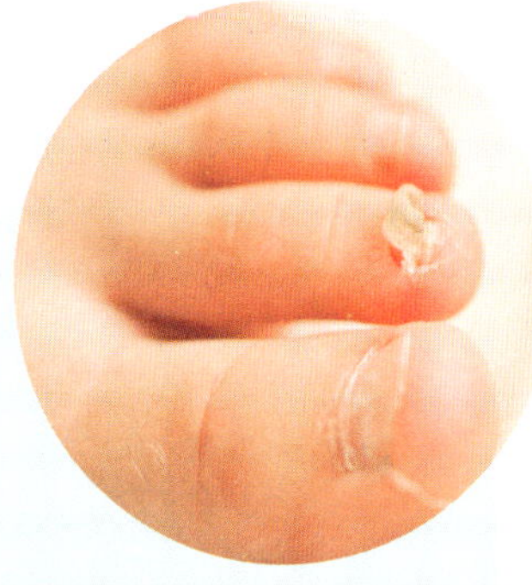

5. **Onychomycosis:** This ringworm infection affects nails – the nail becomes thicker, discoloured and breaks easily.

The typical course of ringworm

Ringworm will usually appear roughly ten days after direct skin-to-skin contact with an infected person, surface or even animal. Be on the lookout for a ring-shaped rash, with itching, scaling and hair loss.

Treatment and management at home

Over-the-counter antifungal creams and sprays can be purchased from any pharmacy, and occasionally oral treatment is needed for tough cases. If you're not sure – or if the rash has not cleared after a week of treatment – have your child seen by a doctor.

Prevention

In general, you can minimise exposure risk by:

1. discouraging the sharing of hairbrushes
2. always wearing footwear in communal showers
3. thoroughly drying certain prone areas after swimming or bathing – like the armpits, groin and in between the toes
4. making sure socks and shoes are clean and dry.

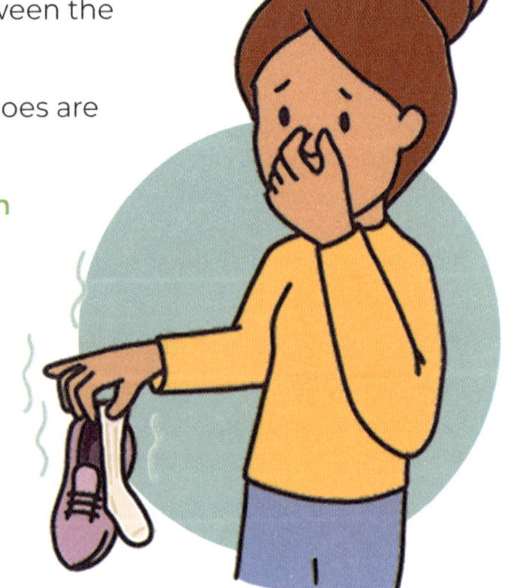

Childcare and school exclusion

Despite ringworm being very infectious, there's no need to exclude your child from childcare or school, as long as you're covering the lesions where possible.

Other gross things

Warts

Have you ever noticed a small, rough bump on your child's skin? It might be a wart, a common and usually harmless skin growth caused by a virus. While a wart might not be the most attractive accessory, there's no need to worry too much. Let's explore what warts are, how they spread and what you can do to help your child.

SYMPTOMS: BUMPY GROWTHS ON HANDS, FEET AND FACE

What is a wart?

Warts are like tiny hitchhikers, catching a ride on the human papillomavirus (HPV). There are many different types of HPV, and some of them like to set up camp on our skin, causing these bumpy growths. Warts can show up anywhere on the body, but they're especially fond of hands, feet and even faces.

How do warts spread?

Warts are often spread through direct contact with another person who has them, or even by touching surfaces that have been in contact with warts.

The typical course of warts

Remember, patience is key when dealing with warts. It can take weeks or even months for them to disappear completely. And while they might seem a bit bothersome, remember that most warts are just temporary visitors that eventually move on.

What are the main types of warts?

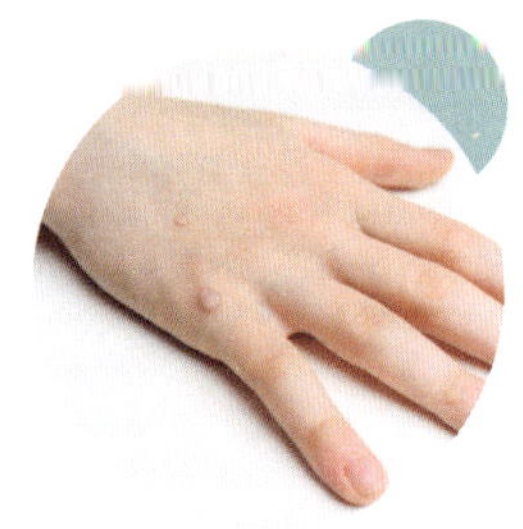

1. **Common warts:** These are the most frequent type, usually appearing on the hands, fingers or knees. They're rough, raised bumps that may have a cauliflower-like appearance.

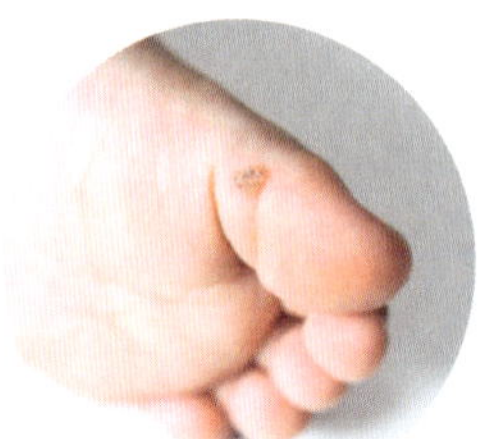

2. **Plantar warts:** These grow on the soles of the feet and can be painful, especially when walking. They often have small black dots in the centre, which are actually tiny blood vessels.

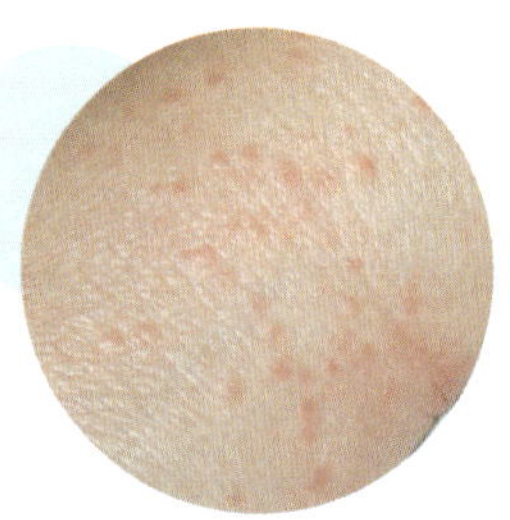

3. **Flat warts:** These are smaller and smoother than common warts and typically appear in clusters on the face, hands or legs.

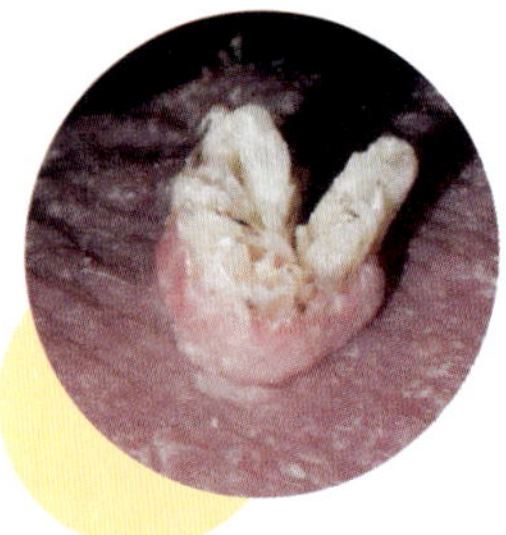

4. **Filiform warts:** These are long, thin warts that usually grow around the mouth, nose or eyes.

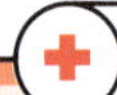

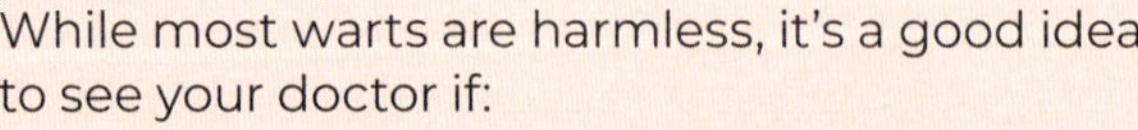

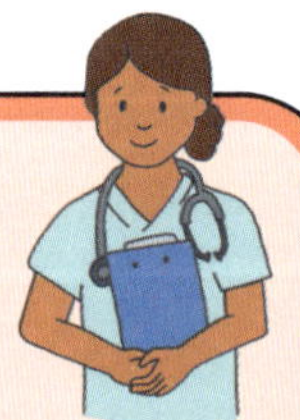

While most warts are harmless, it's a good idea to see your doctor if:

- your child's warts are painful or bleeding
- the warts are spreading rapidly or appear in unusual locations
- your child has a weakened immune system
- you have any ongoing concerns about the warts.

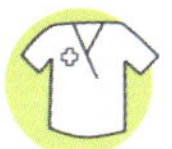

Treatment and management at home

Most warts are completely harmless and often disappear on their own over time, as the body's immune system fights off the virus. However, they can be a bit unsightly and sometimes cause discomfort, especially if they're on the soles of the feet or fingertips.

- Sometimes, simply applying a wart-removal product from the pharmacy can do the trick. These products often contain salicylic acid, which helps to gradually peel away the wart, eventually revealing unblemished skin underneath.
- If the wart is stubborn or causing discomfort, your doctor might recommend other treatments, such as freezing the wart with liquid nitrogen or using a laser. In most cases, these treatments are safe and effective, though they might require multiple sessions.
- **Preparing your child for liquid nitrogen (freezing) and the possible use of a scalpel:** For larger warts that are causing discomfort, I always encourage parents to prepare children by letting them know that the doctor has borrowed a machine from Elsa from *Frozen* to treat their wart. Turning it into a magical ice machine can help alleviate any fear. Reassure them prior to the appointment that sometimes a small knife is used to take the roof off the wart but it doesn't hurt. It's just like getting your hair or nails cut.

Remember: Warts are a common childhood condition that usually resolves over time. With patience and appropriate treatment, you can help your child manage them and reduce the risk of spreading them to others.

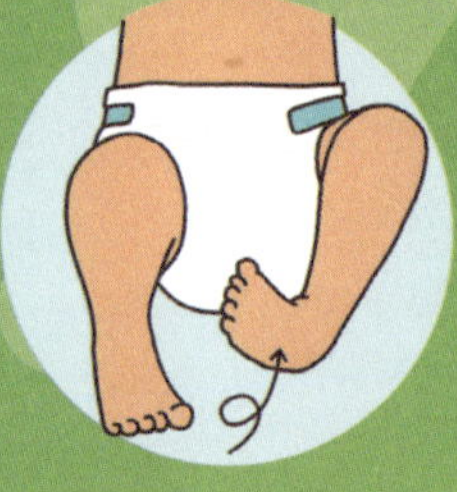

Is this normal?

Club foot pg. 211
Knock knees pg. 213

Is this normal?

Club foot

If your baby has been diagnosed with club foot after birth, it can be a lot to take in. I often meet with families facing this diagnosis, and I want to share some information to help you understand what club foot is, how it's treated, and what you can expect for your child's future.

What is club foot?

Club foot, also called congenital talipes equinovarus (CTEV), is a condition where a baby's foot or feet are turned inward and downward. It happens because the tendons that connect the leg muscles to the foot bones are shorter than usual. While it might look concerning, the good news is that club foot is a very treatable condition.

Club foot should not be confused with positional talipes. This is where a newborn foot displays the same appearance as club foot, but the foot can be moved into the correct position with ease. Positional talipes is caused by the foot being squashed for many months in a contorted position; it usually resolves without any intervention. Talk to your newborn's doctor if you have concerns regarding your child's foot shape or position.

Who does it affect?

Club foot is one of the more common birth differences, affecting about one in a thousand babies. It can affect one or both feet and is more common in boys. It can be detected during a routine pregnancy ultrasound.

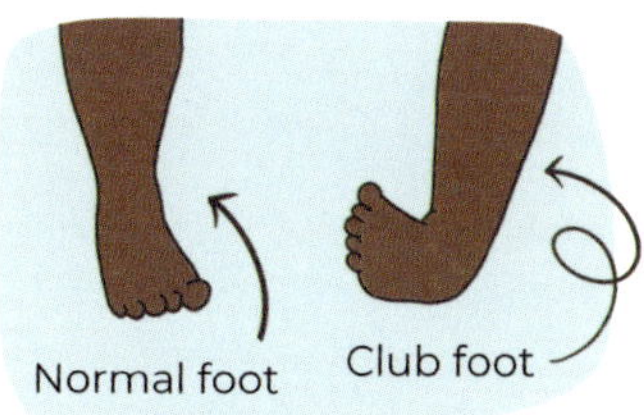

Why does it happen?

We don't always know why club foot occurs. It can be related to the baby's position in the womb, genetics or other factors. What's important to know is that it's not caused by anything a mother did – or didn't do – during pregnancy.

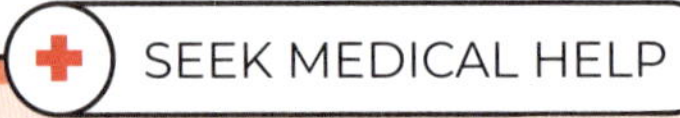

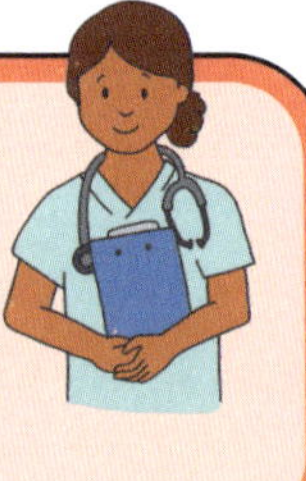

If you notice that your baby's foot or feet appear to be turned inward, it's important to see a doctor, as early treatment leads to the best outcomes.

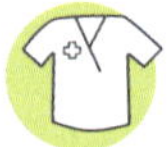

Treatment and management at home

The most common and effective treatment for club foot is the Ponseti method. This involves:

Gentle stretching and casting: Your baby's foot will be gently stretched and placed in a cast to gradually guide it into the correct position. This process is usually repeated weekly for several weeks, stretching the foot further at each visit.

Tenotomy (minor procedure): A small procedure may be needed to lengthen the Achilles tendon at the back of the heel.

Bracing: After the casting is complete, your baby will wear a special brace (usually a bar with shoes attached) to maintain the corrected position and prevent the club foot from returning. The brace is usually worn full-time at first, then gradually for shorter periods over several years.

Common concerns and questions

Will my child be able to walk and run normally?
Absolutely! With proper treatment, most children with club foot go on to walk, run and play just like other kids.

Will my child need surgery?
Surgery is rarely needed, as the Ponseti method is usually enough.

How long will treatment last?
Treatment usually starts soon after birth and continues with bracing for several years.

Can club foot come back?
There's a small chance of recurrence, but it's less likely if the bracing schedule is followed carefully.

Is this normal?

Knock knees

If you've noticed that your child's knees seem to touch when they stand up straight, you might be wondering if it's something to worry about. The answer is usually: no. This condition, called knock knees or genu valgum, is quite common in toddlers and young children.

What are knock knees?

Knock knees are when a child's knees angle inward and touch while their ankles remain apart. It's a little bit like each leg is making a parenthesis shape: **)(** . Knock knees are usually most noticeable between the ages of three and five, and then gradually correct themselves as the child grows.

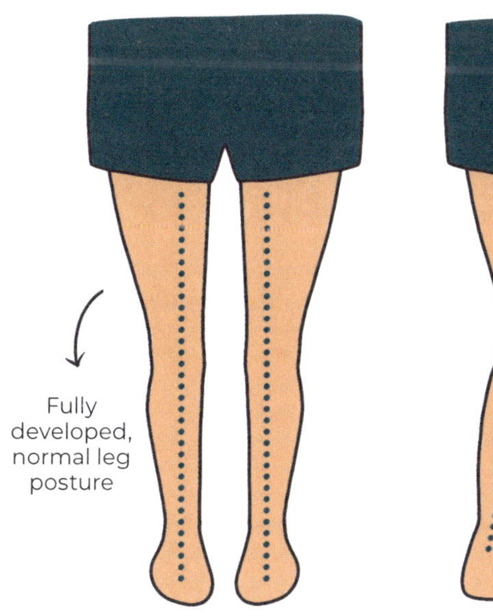

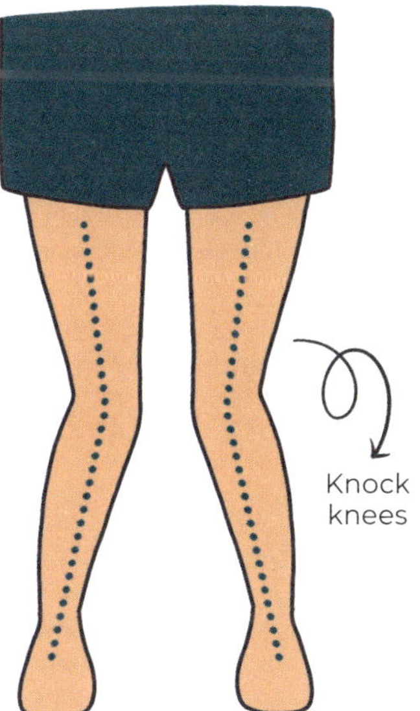

What causes knock knees?

Knock knees are often just a normal part of a child's development. Think of it as a stage their legs go through as their bones and muscles grow and strengthen.

There are a few reasons why it might happen:

- **Ligament laxity:** Young children often have loose ligaments (the tissues that connect bones), which can make their joints more flexible.
- **Growth spurts:** Sometimes, bones grow faster than muscles, which can temporarily affect alignment.
- **Weak muscles:** If the muscles around the knees aren't strong enough, it can lead to knock knees.

Should you be worried?

In most cases, knock knees are nothing to worry about. They usually improve on their own as your child grows and don't cause any pain or problems with walking or running.

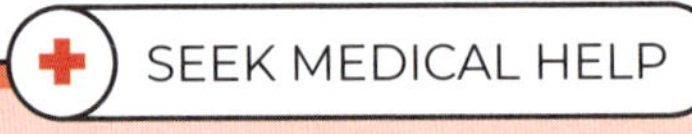

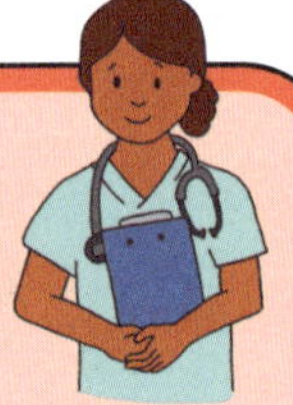

While knock knees usually resolve on their own, consult your doctor if you observe any of the following in your child.

1. **Severe or persistent knock knees:** If your child's knees are very close together or their ankles are far apart, or if knock knees persist beyond the age of seven.

2. **Pain or difficulty walking:** If your child complains of pain or has trouble walking, it's important to see a doctor to rule out any other issues.

3. **One leg is worse than the other:** If knock knees are much more noticeable on one leg than the other.

Serial measurements of the distance between the ankles – when the knees are touching – are a useful way for doctors to monitor the knees over time. If this distance is more than 2.5 cm in children over the age of seven, it suggests knock knees. A gap up to 7 cm is normal between the ages of two and four years.

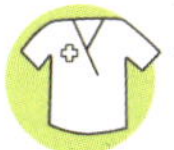

Treatment and management at home

In most cases, you don't need to do anything about knock knees. Your child's legs will naturally straighten out over time. However, there are a few things you can do to support their development:

- **Encourage activity:** Regular exercise helps strengthen the muscles around the knees and promotes healthy bone growth.
- **Promote a healthy diet:** Make sure your child is getting enough calcium and vitamin D for strong bones.
- **Provide proper footwear:** Choose shoes that fit well and provide good support.
- **Avoid 'fixes':** There's no need for special shoes, braces or exercises to correct knock knees. These usually aren't helpful and can even be harmful.

✱ **Remember:** If you have any concerns about your child's knock knees, don't hesitate to talk to your doctor. We can assess your child's development, rule out any underlying conditions, and reassure you if it's just a normal part of growing up.

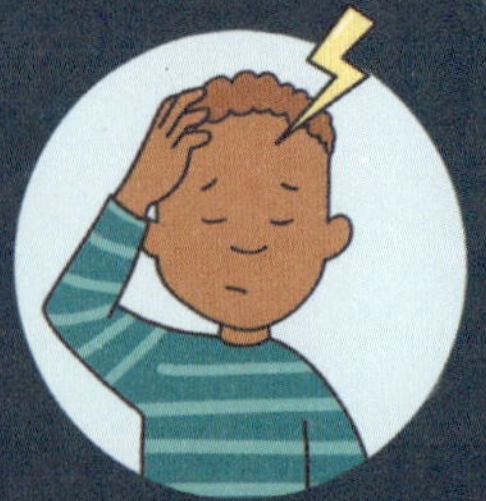

Common medical issues for older kids

Common medical issues for older kids

Headaches

If your child has complained about headaches, they are not alone. Headaches are quite a common complaint in children and teenagers. The reporting of headaches is undeniably difficult in paediatrics. A headache may be reported by children who are tired, dehydrated, bored or defiant, or headaches may represent something more sinister, from poor eyesight to meningitis or raised intracranial pressure (an uncommon medical emergency). Deciphering the origin of a headache is a challenging task.

SYMPTOMS: PAIN OR DISCOMFORT IN THE HEAD OR NECK

What is a headache?

Headaches are basically pain or discomfort in the head or neck region. They can feel like a dull ache, a sharp pain or even pressure.

What are the types of headaches in children?

The most common types of headaches in kids are:

- **Tension headaches:** These feel like a tight band around the head. They can be triggered by stress, fatigue or muscle tension.
- **Migraines:** These are often more severe than tension headaches. They can cause throbbing pain, nausea, vomiting, and sensitivity to light and sound. They tend to be felt down one side of the head or face, and might have a preceding 'aura' or sensory awareness that one is on its way.
- **Other types:** Less common types include cluster headaches, sinus headaches and medication-overuse headaches.

Why do kids get headaches?

Headaches in kids can have many triggers:

1. **Stress:** School pressure, family issues or social anxieties.
2. **Dehydration:** Not drinking enough fluids.
3. **Lack of sleep:** Tiredness can be a major headache trigger.
4. **Certain foods:** Some kids are sensitive to aged cheese, processed meats or artificial sweeteners.
5. **Illness:** Colds, the flu or sinus infections.
6. **Head injury:** A bump on the head can sometimes trigger headaches.
7. **Poor vision or eye strain:** Vision problems can cause headaches, and spending too much time on screens can strain the eyes and lead to headaches, even in the setting of perfect vision.
8. **Puberty:** Migraines are more common in adolescent females entering puberty.

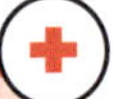

SEEK MEDICAL HELP

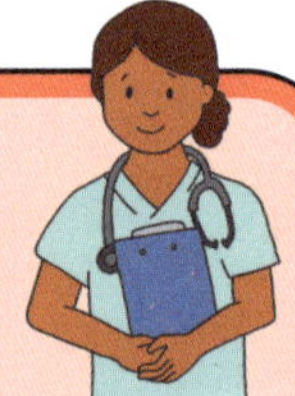

Most headaches in kids are nothing to worry about. However, call your doctor if your child:

- has a sudden, severe headache that comes on quickly
- has a headache that wakes them up from sleep, or recurs in the morning
- has a headache along with a stiff neck, fever or rash
- has a headache after a head injury
- has headaches that are becoming more frequent or severe
- has headaches that interfere with daily life
- has any other symptoms that concern you.

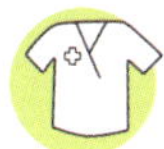

Treatment and management at home

If your child has a headache, try these tips:

- **Rest:** Encourage them to lie down in a quiet, dark room and monitor them regularly.
- **Hydration:** Make sure they drink plenty of fluids.
- **Pain relief:** Over-the-counter pain relievers like ibuprofen or paracetamol may help. Always follow the recommended dosage for your child's age and weight.
- **Relaxation techniques:** Deep breathing, gentle stretching or a warm bath can sometimes help.

Prevention

To help prevent headaches, encourage your child to:

1. **Get enough sleep:** Establish a consistent sleep schedule.
2. **Eat regular meals:** Skipping meals can trigger headaches.
3. **Stay hydrated:** Make sure they drink plenty of water throughout the day.
4. **Manage stress:** Help them find healthy ways to cope with stress.
5. **Limit screen time:** Encourage breaks and outdoor activities.

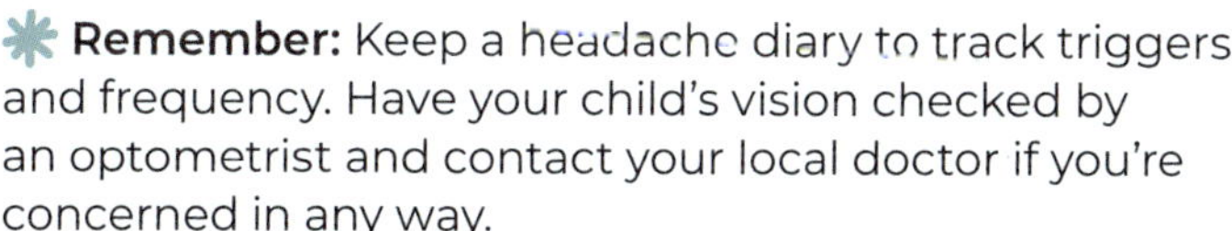

Remember: Keep a headache diary to track triggers and frequency. Have your child's vision checked by an optometrist and contact your local doctor if you're concerned in any way.

Bedwetting

Bedwetting, also known as primary nocturnal enuresis, is something I talk about with families *all the time*. If your child is wetting the bed, know that you're not alone and, most importantly, explain to them that it's nothing to be ashamed of. Remember that new-onset bedwetting in a child who was previously dry overnight, should be investigated by a doctor.

What is bedwetting?

Bedwetting is simply when a child who is old enough to control their bladder urinates during sleep. There are two main types:

1. **Primary enuresis:** The child has never had a consistent period of night-time dryness.
2. **Secondary enuresis:** The child starts wetting the bed after at least six months of dryness.

Remember, toilet-training is a complex interplay between development, hormones and ability. A child can't be trained overnight to stay dry. It's very normal for children who are toilet-trained from an early age during the day to still wet the bed overnight.

Who does it affect?

Bedwetting is more common than you might think! It affects:

- about 15 per cent of five-year-olds
- about 10 per cent of seven-year-olds
- about 3 per cent of twelve-year-olds.

Bedwetting even continues for some teenagers and adults.

As a general rule, I always tell parents to not worry about overnight bedwetting until the child is at school – if they are still wearing overnight nappies when they start primary school, this is a good time to start with simple measures (see below).

I always highlight with my patients that two or three other children in their class will have exactly the same problem they do; this helps to normalise the challenges they face. I also examine the family history; bedwetting is a highly inherited condition, so if your child sees that you, too, faced this challenge as a child, they will more easily see themselves growing out of it.

Why does it happen?

There are a few reasons why bedwetting occurs:

- **Bladder size:** Some children have smaller bladders that fill up more quickly.
- **Hormones:** A hormone called anti-diuretic hormone (ADH) helps concentrate urine overnight. Some kids don't produce enough ADH, so they make larger volumes of urine.
- **Deep sleep:** Some children are such deep sleepers that they don't wake up when their bladder is full. It's always important to use positive language around this, and explain to children that they wet the bed because they are SUCH a great sleeper. Avoid using terms like 'accidents' when bedwetting occurs.
- **Constipation:** This can put pressure on the bladder, limiting how much urine it can store overnight.
- **Medical conditions:** Rarely, bedwetting can be a sign of an underlying medical condition, like a urinary tract infection or diabetes.
- **Stress or anxiety:** Although largely anecdotal, many children experience an increase in bedwetting when stressed (whether physically or emotionally).
- **Changes in routine:** A holiday house with an unfamiliar route to the toilet may be the simplest of explanations for new-onset bedwetting. Similarly, changes in time zones or routines when on holidays can lead to unexpected bedwetting.

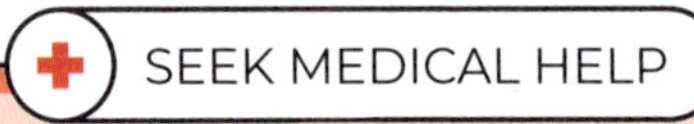

Talk to your doctor if:

- bedwetting is causing your child distress or affecting their self-esteem
- bedwetting starts suddenly after a period of dryness
- you notice any other symptoms, like pain during urination, increased thirst or constipation.

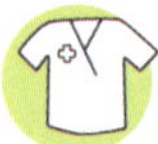

Treatment and management at home

There are several effective treatments for bedwetting, but avoid rushing to a solution in young children. Normalise it as much as possible, and only implement treatments when it becomes a problem *for the child.*

Bedwetting tips:

- Limit fluid intake before bedtime and improve daytime hydration.
- Encourage your child to use the toilet right before bed.
- Treat constipation (if present).
- **Bedwetting alarms:** These alarms wake the child up when they start to urinate, helping them learn to recognise the sensation of a full bladder. Over a course of two months, they are effective in over 85 per cent of children.
- **Medications:** There are a few medications that can be helpful for some children, though these should be used sparingly, i.e. for sleepovers or school camps.

Other practical tips for bedwetting

TIP 1:

Offer your child a toilet visit at 10–10.30 pm after gently waking them. Slightly rouse your child and take them to the toilet. Often, most children won't even remember going to the toilet with you but it can help them last through until the morning and, as they haven't fully woken, they should return to deep sleep fairly quickly.

TIP 2:
Ensure your child drinks consistently and evenly over the day so they are well hydrated.

TIP 3:
Don't use punishment if they do wet the bed overnight. NEVER scold or yell at them, as it is never a behavioural issue (never by choice). Kids have to be ready to be toilet-trained overnight, and punishing them will not make this happen any faster.

TIP 4:
If you're worried they might be resisting going to the toilet at night because they're too cold, keep their room a little warmer.

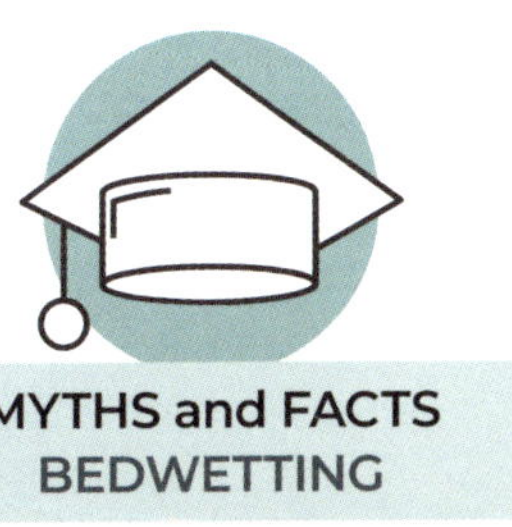

MYTHS and FACTS
BEDWETTING

Myth: Punishing or shaming a child will stop bedwetting.

Fact: Punishing a child for bedwetting can make the problem worse by increasing stress and anxiety.

Myth: Bedwetting is a sign of laziness or emotional problems.

Fact: Bedwetting is a medical condition, not a behavioural one. It's not your child's fault; they are not being lazy or doing this on purpose.

Myth: Bedwetting will always go away on its own.

Fact: While many children outgrow bedwetting, some need a little extra help.

Remember: Be patient and supportive. Never reprimand overnight bedwetting; positive reinforcement is the key. Celebrate dry nights! Don't hesitate to seek help but don't set unrealistic expectations. Bedwetting is a common and treatable problem.

Breath-holding spells

If you've ever witnessed a child having a breath-holding spell, you know how frightening it can be, and I understand the worry it can cause. The good news is that breath-holding spells, while scary to watch, are usually harmless and something children outgrow.

What are breath-holding spells?

A breath-holding spell is when a child involuntarily stops breathing for a short period, usually just a few seconds. It can happen when a child is upset, frustrated, angry or in pain. Sometimes, they might even faint briefly or have involuntary movements.

There are two main types:

1. **Cyanotic breath-holding spells:** The child's face turns blue or purple. These usually happen when the child is upset or frustrated and starts crying, then suddenly after an inhalation, a cry or exhalation is withheld, and the child pauses breathing.

2. **Pallid breath-holding spells:** The child's face turns pale or white. These often occur after a sudden fright, from pain or a big surprise.

Why do breath-holding spells happen?

The exact cause of breath-holding spells isn't fully understood. It's believed to be a reflex, a bit like a hiccough, that some children are more prone to. There seems to be a genetic component, as breath-holding spells sometimes run in families. Breath-holding spells are *not* an attention-seeking behaviour and are not a form of epilepsy (seizure syndrome).

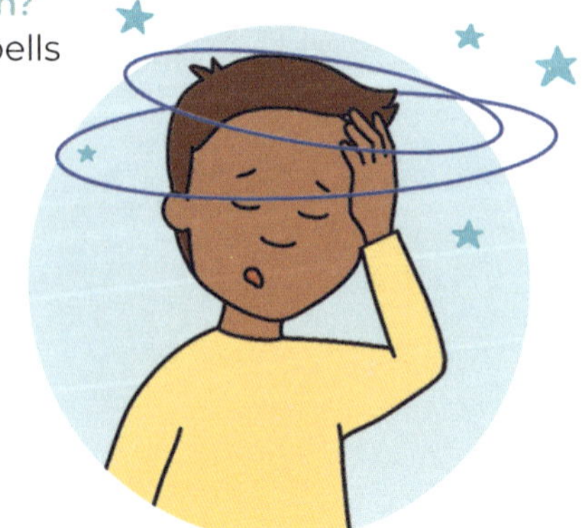

Are breath-holding spells dangerous?

While they are alarming for parents to witness, breath-holding spells are generally not dangerous. The child's breathing always returns on its own, and the spells don't cause any lasting harm. It's important to know that breath-holding spells are NOT related to seizures or epilepsy. The biggest danger in a breath-holding spell is actually the risk of a child bumping their head from a faint.

What to do during a breath-holding spell

1. **Stay calm:** I know it's easier said than done, but staying calm is the most important thing you can do. Otherwise, your child will pick up on your anxiety.

2. **Let it pass:** Don't try to force your child to breathe or shake them. The spell will resolve on its own within a minute.

3. **Safety first:** If your child faints, gently lay them on their side on a soft surface to prevent injury from falls.

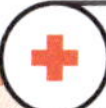

SEEK MEDICAL HELP

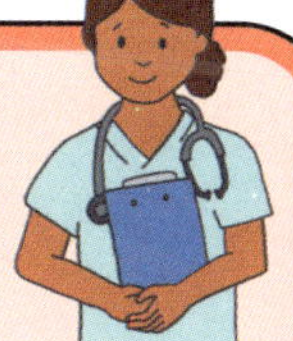

Most breath-holding spells don't require medical attention. However, consult your local doctor if:

- your child experiences their first episode
- your child is having more than one spell a week
- the spells last longer than a minute
- your child seems to be recovering slowly from the spells
- the spell involves significant shaking movements (seizure activity)
- you have any other concerns about your child's health.

Prevention

While there's no guaranteed way to prevent breath-holding spells, here are a few tips that might help:

- **Identify triggers:** If you notice patterns (like spells always happening when your child is frustrated), try to address the underlying cause. Behaviour modification plans are helpful here.
- **Stay calm:** Your calm demeanour can help your child learn to manage their emotions better.
- **Use positive reinforcement:** Reward your child for staying calm and managing their feelings without having a spell.
- **Check iron levels:** Iron-deficiency anaemia is more common in children with breath-holding spells, so your doctor may request a blood test to check iron levels and consider starting an iron supplement.

Remember: You are not alone. Breath-holding spells are more common than you might think. Your child will outgrow them. Most children stop having breath-holding spells by the age of five or six. Talk to your paediatrician if you have any concerns.

Common medical issues for older kids

Snoring

Snoring is surprisingly common in children, and while it can be cute (and sometimes a little funny), it's important to understand what it means and when it might be a sign of something more sinister.

Why do children snore?

Snoring happens when the airway (the passage for air to travel in and out of the lungs) becomes partially blocked during sleep. This obstruction causes the tissues in the airway to vibrate, creating that familiar snoring sound. In children, snoring can be caused by a variety of different factors:

1. **Enlarged tonsils and adenoids:** These are tissues in the back of the throat and nasal passages that can become enlarged due to allergies, infections or other reasons.
2. **Turbinate hypertrophy:** Probably the most under-appreciated cause of disrupted sleep. Turbinates are small, bony projections (covered in gland tissue) in the nose. Enlarged turbinates promote mouth-breathing, which can lead to snoring.
3. **Allergies or colds:** Congestion and inflammation can narrow the airway, making snoring more likely during an episode of illness or allergy.
4. **Obesity:** Extra weight around the neck can put pressure on the airway.
5. **Deviated septum:** The septum is the wall that divides the nasal passages. If it's crooked (deviated), it can obstruct airflow and cause snoring.
6. **Sleep apnoea:** This is a more serious condition in which breathing repeatedly stops and starts during sleep. Snoring is a common symptom of sleep apnoea.
7. **Pillow:** Inappropriate pillow size can cause awkward head posturing and put pressure on the airway.

SEEK MEDICAL HELP

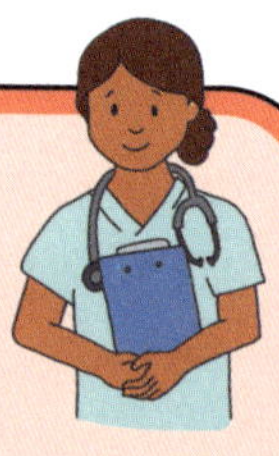

Occasional snoring, especially if it's mild and your child seems well-rested, is usually not a cause for concern. However, you should talk to your local doctor if your child's snoring is:

- **Frequent:** Happening most nights.
- **Loud:** Loud enough to be heard through closed doors.
- **Disruptive:** Wakes your child or disturbs their sleep.
- **Accompanied by other symptoms:** Gasping or choking sounds during sleep, daytime sleepiness, behavioural problems, concentration/focus difficulties or poor growth. These could be signs of a more serious condition like obstructive sleep apnoea, which can have long-term consequences if left untreated.

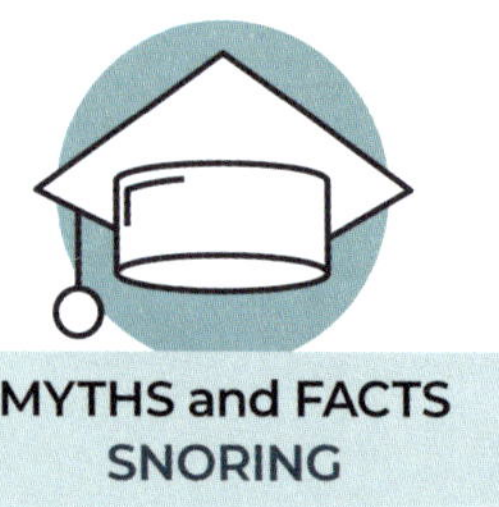

MYTHS and FACTS
SNORING

Myth: Children will outgrow snoring.

Fact: While some children do outgrow snoring, others don't, especially if there's an underlying cause like enlarged tonsils, turbinate hypertrophy or sleep apnoea.

Myth: Snoring is always harmless in children.

Fact: While usually benign, snoring can sometimes be a sign of an underlying issue that needs attention. Persistent snoring in children should always be investigated (and in adults too).

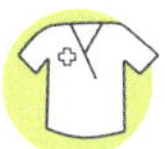 Treatment and management at home

If your child snores, the first step is to talk to your doctor or paediatrician. We can assess your child's overall health, examine their airway, and determine if any further evaluation is needed.

Depending on the cause, treatment options might include:

- **Lifestyle changes:** If obesity is a factor, a healthy diet and increased activity can be helpful. Sometimes a simple review of your child's pillow can change their sleep quality entirely!
- **Allergy management:** If allergies are contributing, managing them with trigger avoidance or medications can improve snoring.
- **Medications:** In some cases, nasal sprays or other medications can help reduce congestion and improve airflow.
- **Surgery:** If enlarged tonsils, adenoids or turbinates are the cause, surgery might be recommended.

 **Remember:**

Be observant: pay attention to your child's snoring patterns and any associated symptoms.

Don't hesitate to ask questions: talk to your doctor if you have any concerns about your child's snoring or sleep quality.

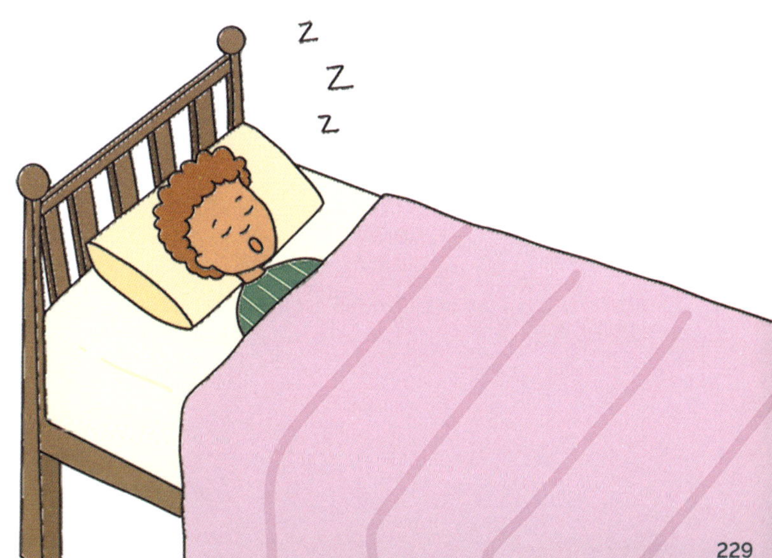

Acne

If your child or teenager is dealing with acne, it can be a frustrating and sometimes embarrassing experience. Acne is one of the most common skin conditions in both children and adolescents – somewhat of a rite of passage.

SYMPTOMS: PIMPLES, BLACKHEADS, WHITEHEADS

What is acne?

Acne vulgaris is a skin condition that occurs when hair follicles become clogged with oil and dead skin cells. This can lead to the formation of pimples, blackheads, whiteheads and, in more severe cases, even deeper lumps (cysts or nodules).

What's the difference between acne and pimples?

Acne is a disease. Pimples may be a symptom of acne.

What are the types of pimples?

With acne, there are many types of pimples, and the symptoms depend on which kind you have.

These include:

- **Papules** are mostly flat, but can become inflamed (tender and warm to touch).
- Comedone is the medical term for a follicle blocked by oil and dead skin. Open comedones are **blackheads** (due to surface pigment, not dirt) and closed comedones are **whiteheads**, where the follicle is completely blocked.
- **Nodules** are larger, irregular-shaped masses. They are usually under the skin surface and may cause pain or discomfort.

- **Pustules** look like whiteheads with a surrounding red ring. Interfering with pustules (by squeezing or popping) can lead to permanent scars.
- Similarly, **cysts** are pimples filled with a thick yellow or white fluid containing bacteria and dead cells (pus). Interfering with cysts can also cause scars.

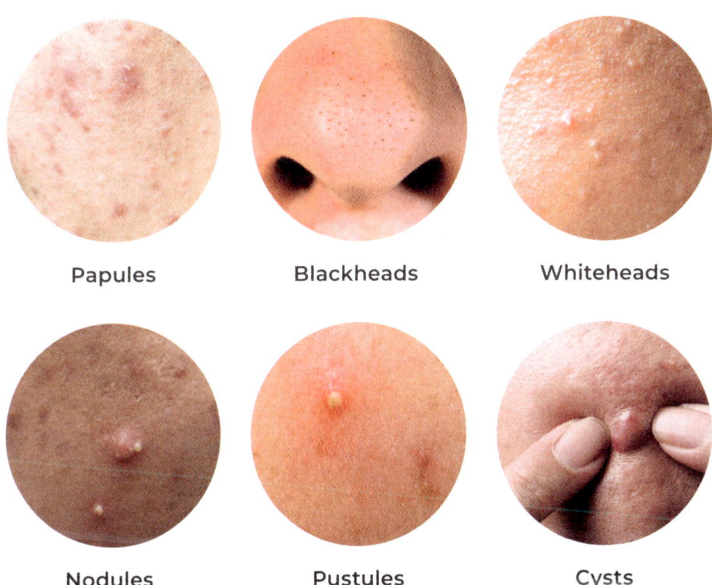

Papules Blackheads Whiteheads

Nodules Pustules Cysts

Why do children and teens get acne?

Several factors contribute to acne development, and these are often amplified during puberty:

1. **Hormones:** Increased levels of hormones called androgens can trigger excess oil production, leading to clogged pores.
2. **Genetics:** If you or your partner had acne, your child is more likely to develop it.
3. **Bacteria:** A bacterium called *Cutibacterium acnes* (sounds cute but certainly isn't) thrives in clogged pores and can contribute to inflammation.
4. **Friction or irritation:** Things like tight clothing, fringes, helmets or backpacks can irritate the skin and worsen acne.
5. **Certain medications:** Some medications, like corticosteroids or lithium, can trigger acne.

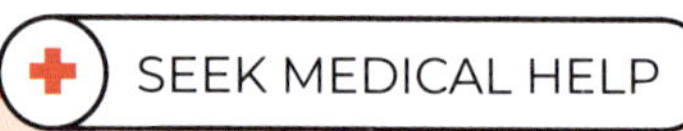

If your child's acne is causing them distress, or if over-the-counter treatments aren't working, it's time to see a doctor. We can help develop a treatment plan tailored to your child's specific needs.

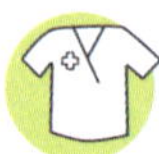

Treatment and management at home

The good news is that there are many effective treatments for acne. Here are some options:

- **Over-the-counter products:** Look for cleansers and creams containing benzoyl peroxide, salicylic acid or adapalene. These can help unclog pores and reduce inflammation.
- **Prescription medications:** If over-the-counter products aren't working, your doctor may prescribe stronger creams or oral antibiotics.
- **Other treatments:** In more severe cases, treatments like oral contraceptives (for girls), isotretinoin medications or light therapy might be considered.

Resisting the urge to 'pop' a pimple
While my strong and consistent advice is to avoid the urge to pop or squeeze pimples and let them heal on their own, many of us know the temptation is often too much. If your adolescent is going to pop a pimple and remove the pus from a whitehead or squeeze a blackhead, it's incredibly important that they do so in a sterile way.

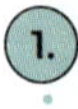

Apply a hot compress. A hot compress can soothe the pain of a pimple that's inflamed. Once pores are opened by applying heat, your pimple may be able to open and release on its own.

2. Pop the pimple in a sterile way, if you must!

Step 1:

Wash and cleanse the face.

Step 2:

Steam your skin.

- Use a face steamer or a hot bowl of water with a towel over your head.
- Relax for ten minutes.

Step 3:

Wash your hands and/or put on surgical gloves.

Step 4:

Wipe the site with an alcohol swab.

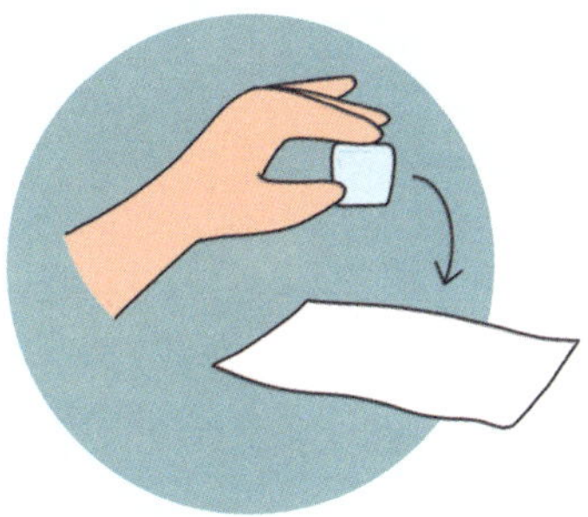

Step 5:

Using cotton pads on either side of the pimple, use your index fingers to gently press down.

- If it isn't easily popped after five seconds, it's not ready, and forcing it may damage your skin.
- Never squeeze so hard that you draw blood.

Step 6:

Wash and cleanse your face again.

Step 7:

Consider using ice to reduce swelling. Wrap an ice cube in a clean cloth or paper towel, and ice the site for one minute to help with any swelling or inflammation.

Step 8:

Remember that your paediatrician said not to squeeze it in the first place!

Preferred method for blackheads

Follow steps 1–4 from previous page. Rather than using cotton pads, use your index fingers (not the nails) to press inward and down on the blackhead. Avoid squeezing too close to the blackhead, as it will make it harder to remove.

Pimples you should never pop

There are some types of pimples that you should never try to pop, including:

1. **Any red pimple without a white head:** These pimples are not yet close enough to the surface of the skin to be drained.
2. **Big, inflamed, deep blemishes:** These could be nodular breakouts or cysts. You should never squeeze this type of acne because the core of the pimple is too deep in the skin. It's best to let them heal on their own.
3. **A large and very painful blemish:** You might think these are just big pimples, but they could actually be boils. See your doctor.

Make-up will make it worse: Many adolescents apply foundation or make-up to cover acne; this almost always worsens the problem and should be discouraged.

Acne can have a huge impact on your child's self-esteem, confidence and general mental health, and they might need a little more TLC and understanding from you as their parent and number-one support.

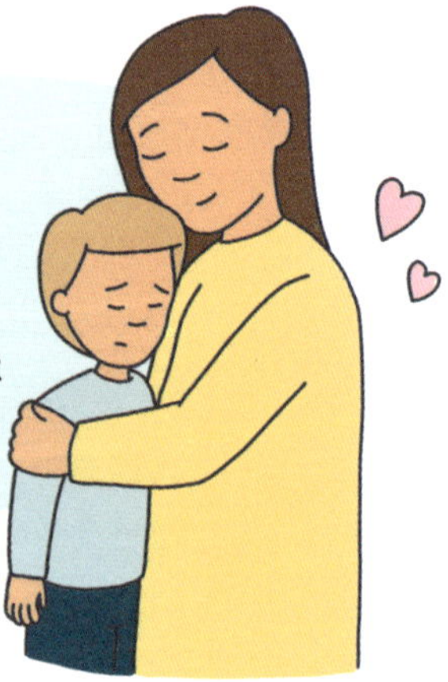

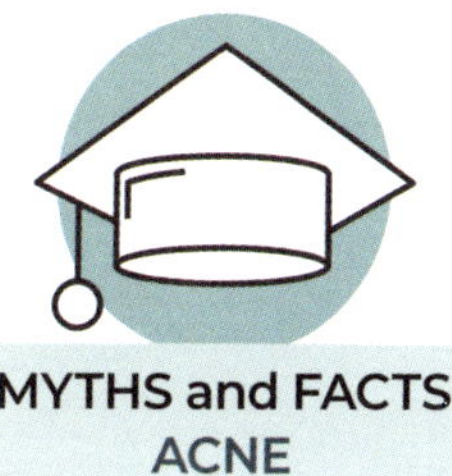

MYTHS and FACTS ACNE

Myth: Acne is caused by poor hygiene.

Fact: While regular washing is important, over-washing or using harsh products can irritate the skin and make acne worse.

Myth: Certain foods cause acne.

Fact: The link between diet and acne is still being researched, but there's no strong evidence that specific foods like chocolate or greasy food directly cause acne. Still, a healthy, balanced diet is always a good idea for overall health and wellbeing.

Myth: Popping pimples will make them go away faster.

Fact: Popping pimples can push bacteria deeper into the skin and increase inflammation, potentially leading to more breakouts, infections, pits and scarring. The pustule is actually keeping the bacteria nice and contained. Left alone, a blemish will heal itself in a few days. Popped improperly, it can linger for weeks or lead to complications.

 **Remember:**

Be patient: acne treatments often take time to work; in the meantime encourage your child to try to avoid make-up and foundation.

Be gentle: encourage your child to avoid scrubbing or picking at pimples.

Don't compare: everyone's skin is different. What works for one person might not work for another.

Talk to your child: reassure them that acne is common and treatable.

Quick reference

Childcare and school exclusion

Condition	Childcare and school exclusion cases	Page
Blocked tear ducts	Exclusion is not necessary.	182
Bronchiolitis	Exclude until well.	92
Chickenpox	Exclude until all blisters have dried. This is usually at least five days after the rash appears in unimmunised children, but may be less in previously immunised children.	128
Cold sores	Young children unable to comply with good hygiene practices should be excluded while the lesion is weeping. Lesions should be covered by a dressing, where possible.	136
Common cold	Exclude until well.	76
Conjunctivitis	Exclude until discharge from eyes has ceased.	179
COVID-19	Exclude until well.	114
Croup	Exclude until well.	100
Ear infection	Exclusion is not necessary.	175
Gastro	In an outbreak of gastroenteritis, exclude until there has been no vomiting or loose bowel motions for forty-eight hours. For all other diarrhoeal illnesses, exclude until there has been no vomiting or loose bowel motions for twenty-four hours.	71
HFMD	Exclude until all blisters have dried.	124
Head lice	Exclude until the day after treatment has commenced.	196
Influenza	Exclude until well.	96

Condition	Childcare and school exclusion cases	Page
Measles	Exclude for at least four days after onset of rash. Unimmunised contacts should be excluded until fourteen days after the first appearance of rash in the initial case.	140
Meningococcal disease	Exclude until adequate carrier eradication therapy has been completed.	144
Molluscum	Exclusion is not necessary.	157
Pinworms	Exclusion is not necessary.	189
Pneumonia	Exclude until well.	107
Ringworm (tinea)	Exclude until the day after treatment has commenced.	204
RSV	Exclude until well.	88
Scabies	Exclude until the day after treatment has commenced.	161
School sores (impetigo)	Exclude until treatment has commenced. Sores on exposed surfaces must be covered with a watertight dressing.	153
Slapped cheek	Exclude for twenty-four hours *after* the fever has resolved.	132
Sepsis	Exclude until well.	171
Strep throat	Exclude until the child has received antibiotic treatment for at least twenty-four hours and the child feels well.	104
Whooping cough (pertussis)	Exclude the child for twenty-one days after the onset of cough or until they have completed five days of a course of antibiotics.	110

Quick reference

Rash

Acne (adolescent)
p. 230-1

Blackheads
p. 230-1

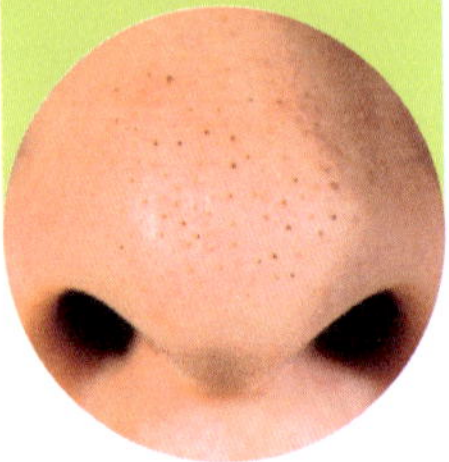

Whiteheads
p. 230-1

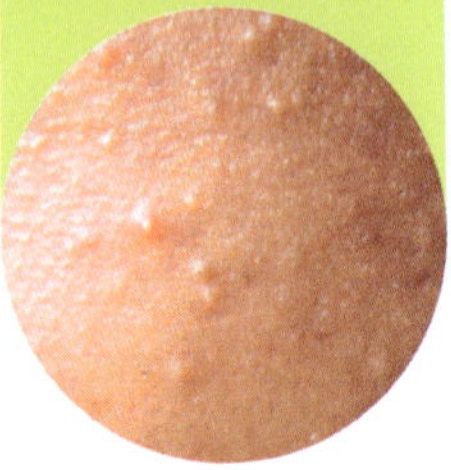

Papules
p. 230-1

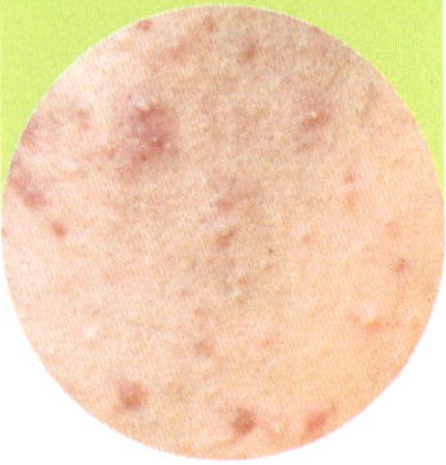

Pustules
p. 230-1

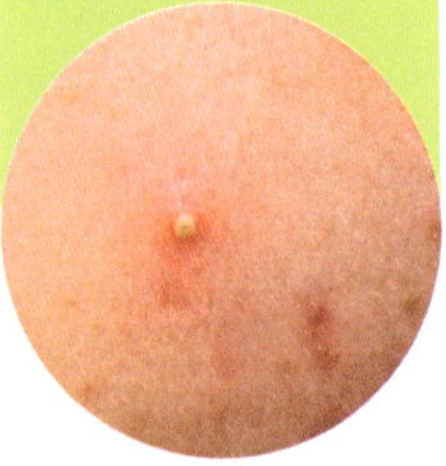

Nodules
p. 230-1

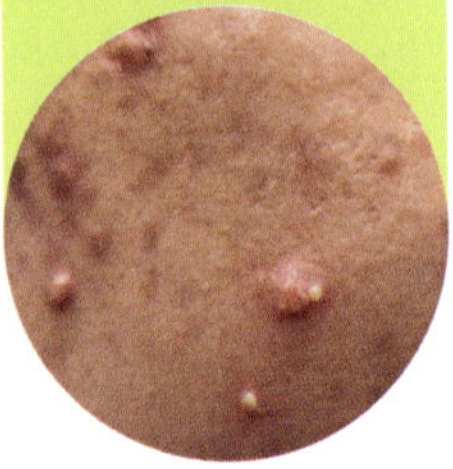

Cysts
p. 230-1

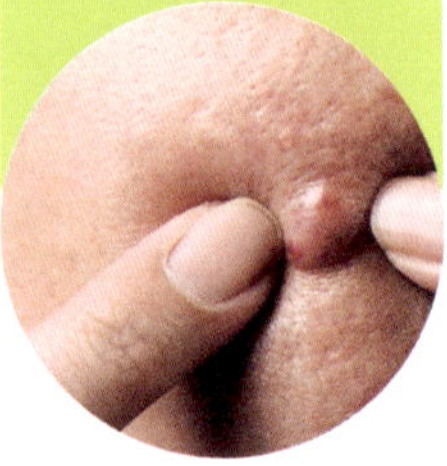

Acne (newborn)
p. 230-1

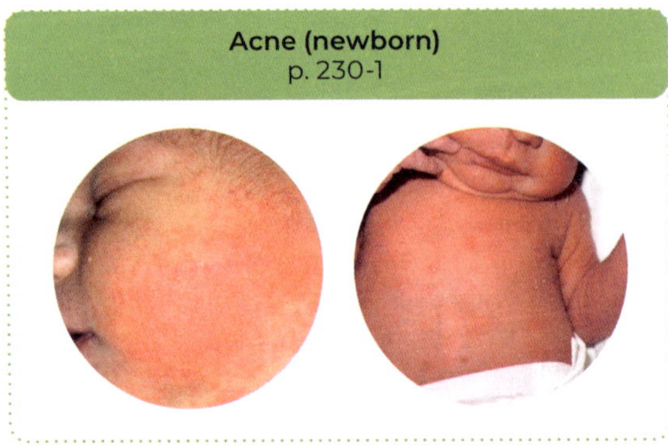

Chickenpox

p. 128

Cold sores

p. 136

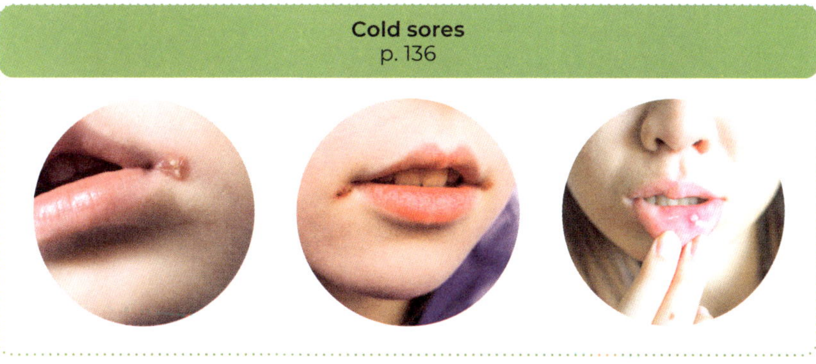

Cutis marmorata

Eczema

p. 164

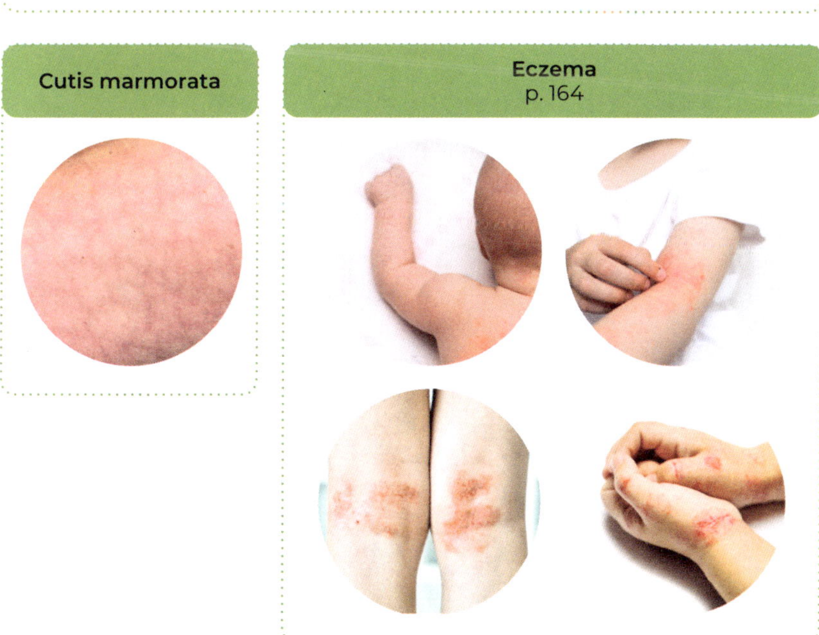

HFMD: hand, foot and mouth disease
p. 124

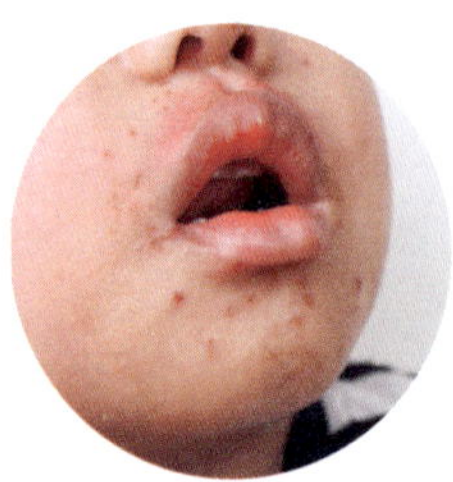

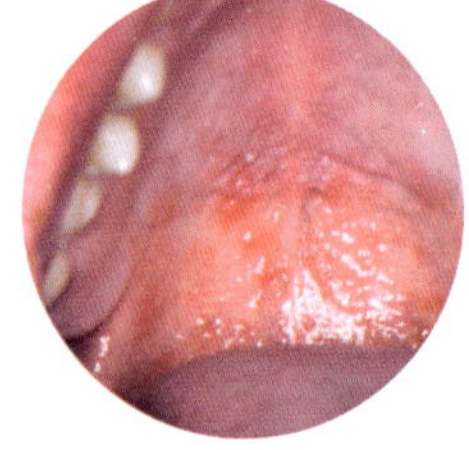

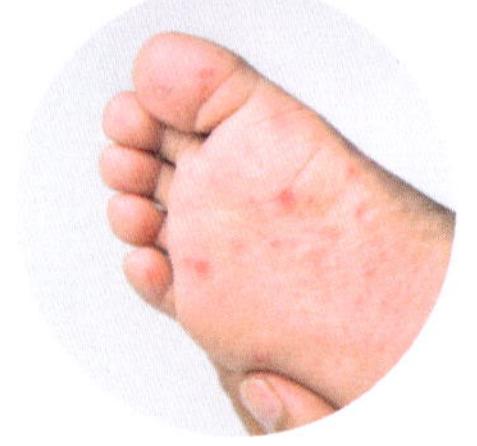

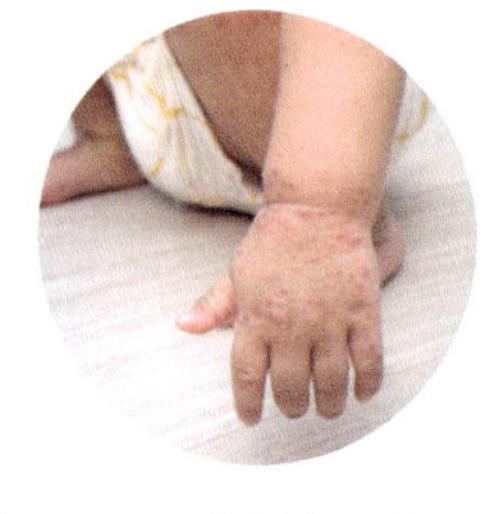

Hives
Hives (or urticaria) are a skin rash involving raised, itchy welts on the skin. These are typically red but may also be skin coloured.

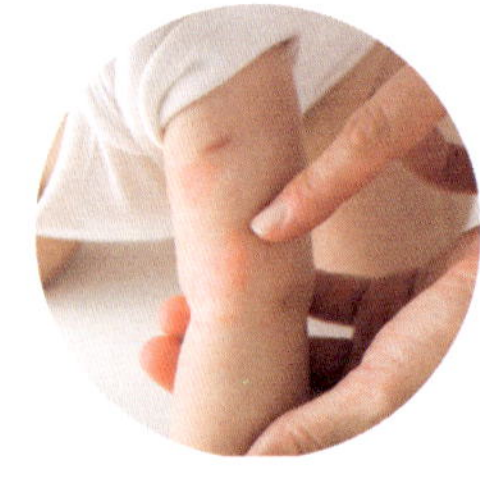

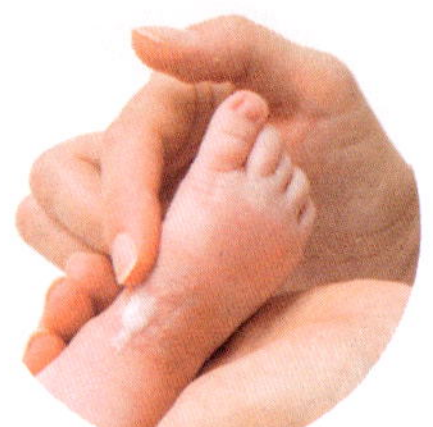

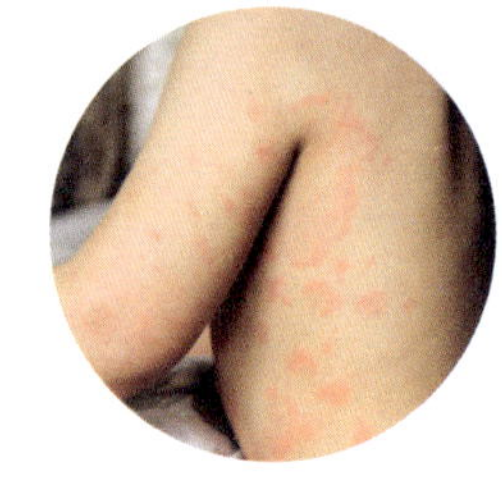

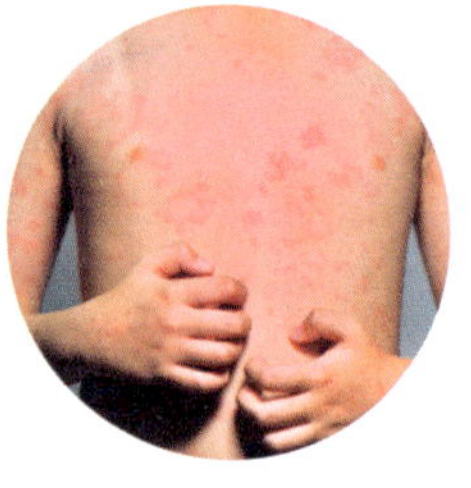

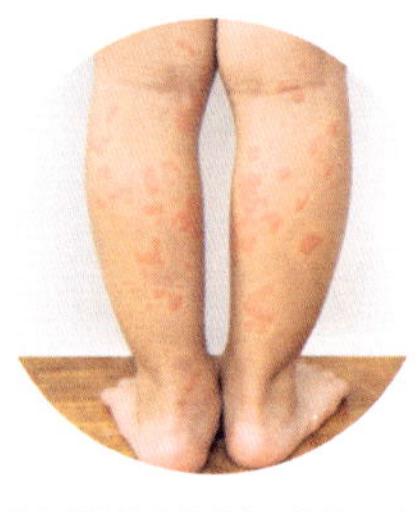

HSP: Henoch-Schönlein purpura
p. 150

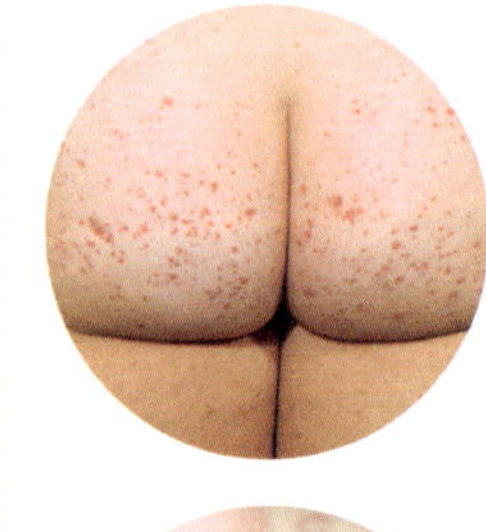

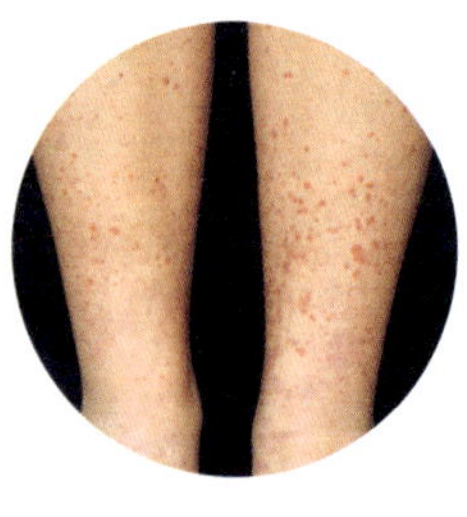

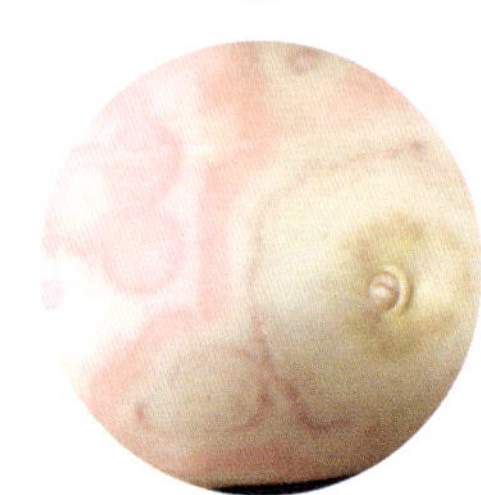

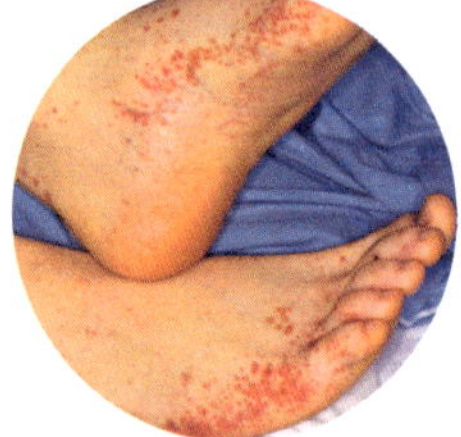

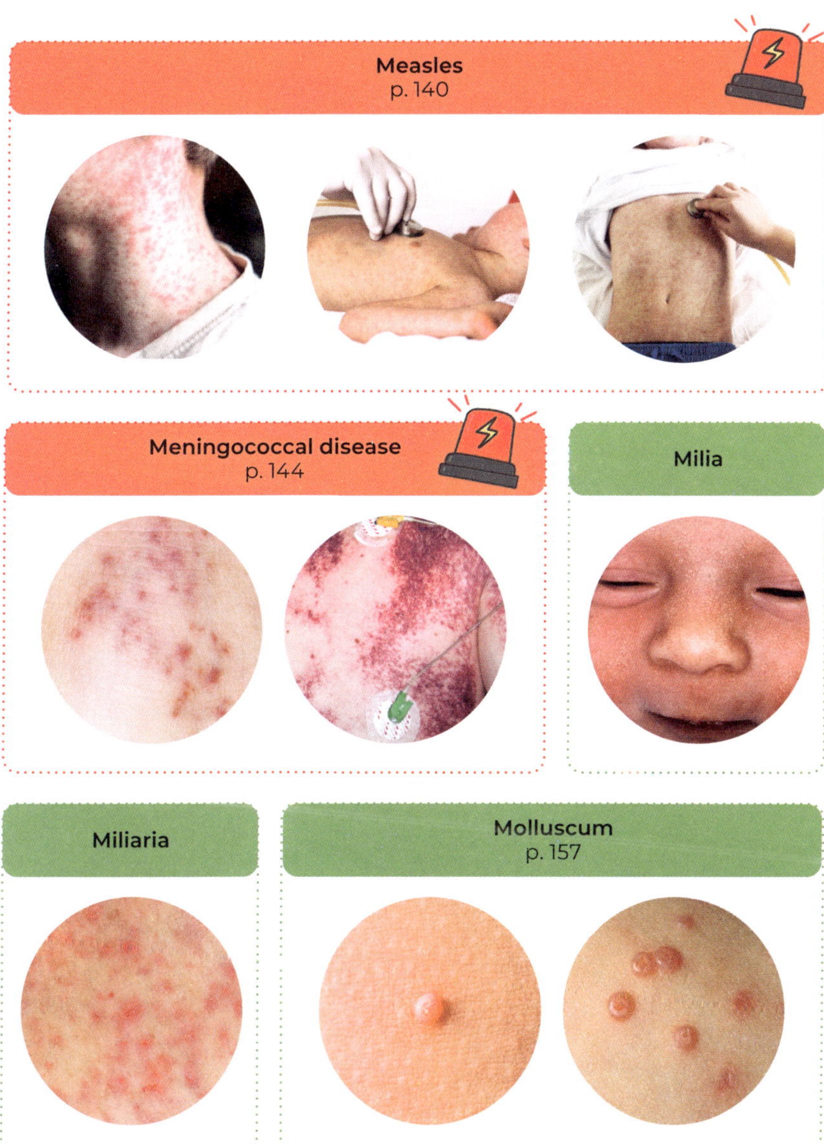
Measles
p. 140
Meningococcal disease
p. 144
Milia
Miliaria
Molluscum
p. 157

Nappy rash

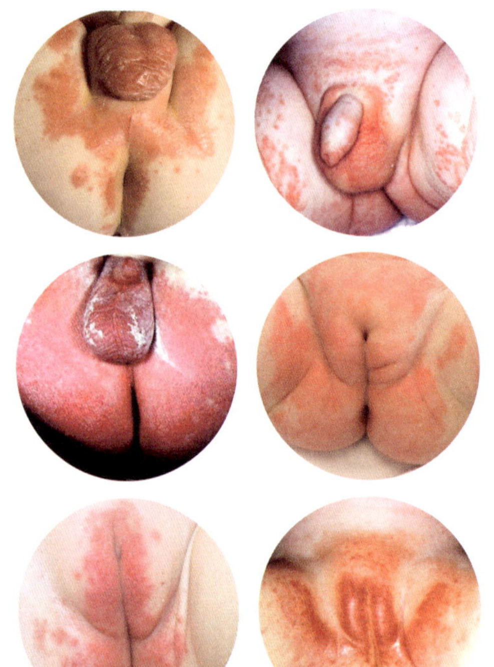

Roseola infantum

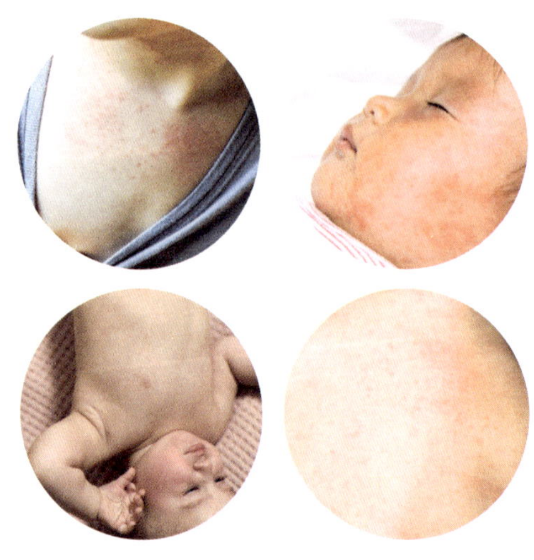

Scabies

p.160

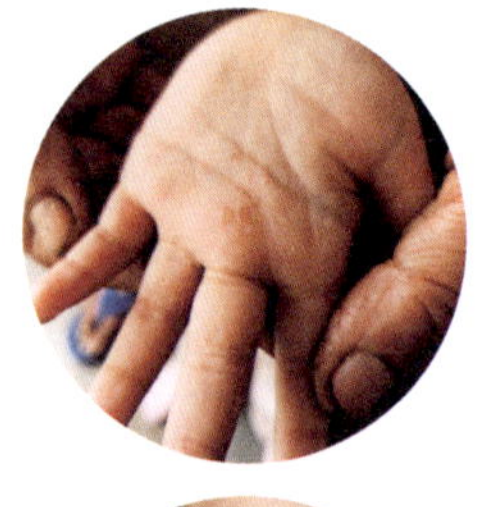

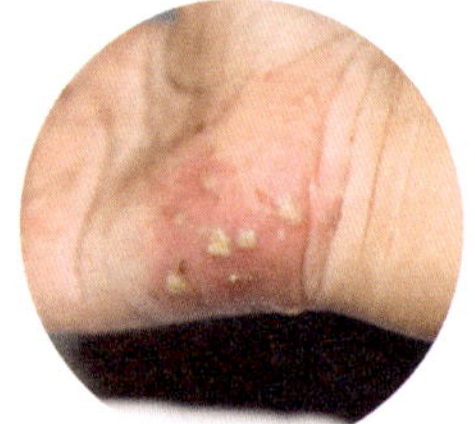

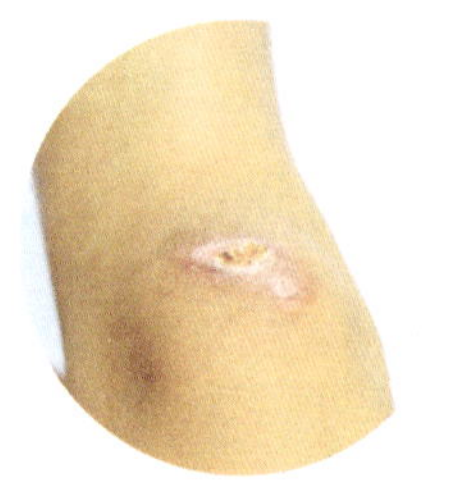

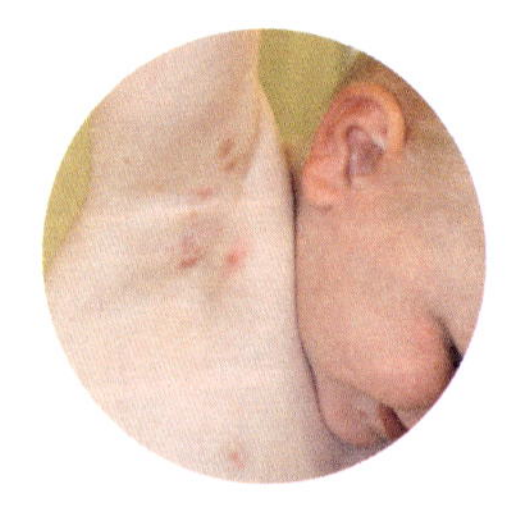

School sores (impetigo)

p. 153

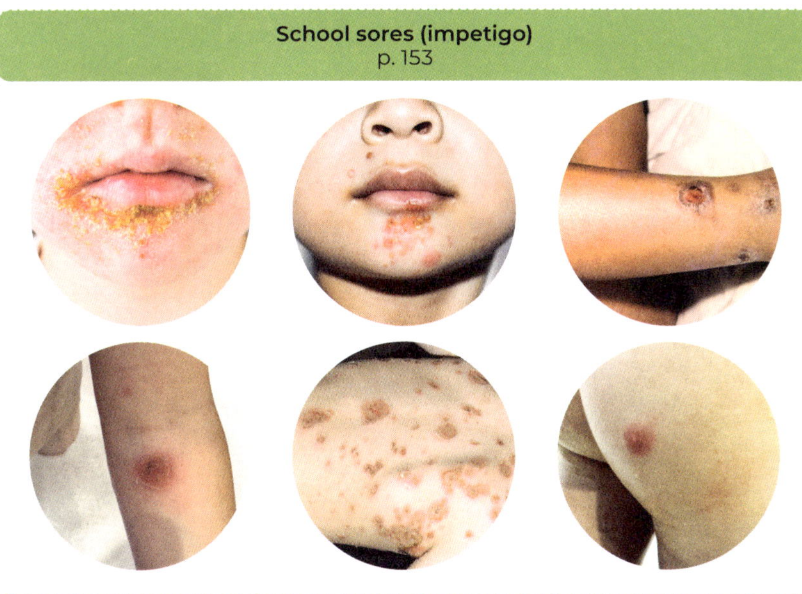

Slapped cheek

p. 132

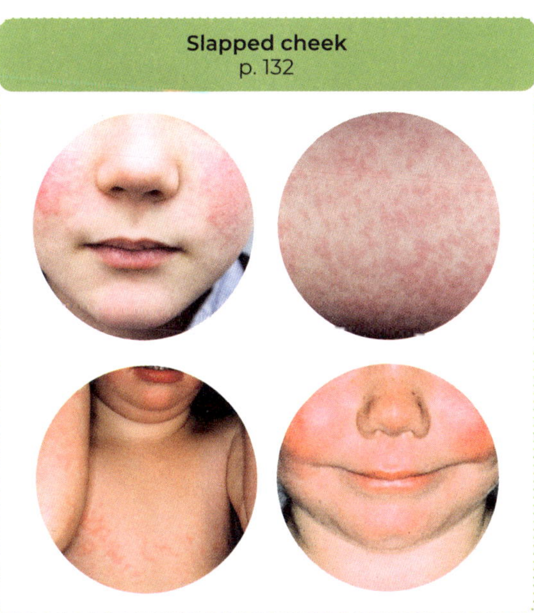

What I always want you to remember as parents

The health and wellbeing of our family are perhaps THE MOST important things we must protect as parents.

At the start of this book we discussed:

1. **Using the medical system when needed.** It's here to help you and your family. I urge you to understand the resources you have access to, and have contact details readily accessible. Never hesitate to utilise these services when required.

2. **Trusting your parental instincts.** This sixth sense is seldom ever wrong. If you're worried, always back yourself. No one knows your child better than you.

This book is your quick-reference guide when it comes to common childhood illnesses. It does not replace medical care. No matter what the condition or illness may be, if you suspect something isn't quite right with your child, have them reviewed by a healthcare professional.

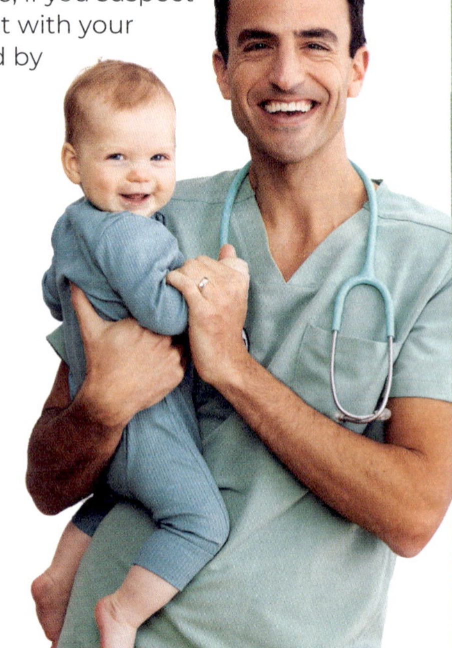

As a parent, you will undoubtedly navigate through some of the conditions covered in this book. It is designed to empower you with the confidence to discern normal from abnormal, and what needs emergency care from things that can be managed safely at home.

I truly hope it helps your family.

Author acknowledgements

Thank you to everyone who has contributed to, and reviewed, this book. To the publishing and editing team at Hardie Grant Children's Publishing: what an extraordinary group you are. Alannah, you've been on this journey every step of the way and to say that none of this would have been possible without you is an understatement. Cora, you are a wonder, and you have brought this book to life. To Dr Joe Spencer and Dr Natasha Ching: your collective expertise has been invaluable.

To my wife and children, thank you for teaching, rewarding, challenging and fulfilling me, every single day. To the thousands of families who have joined the Dr Golly Sleep Program and follow me across platforms, I thank you for your ongoing support. I am so thrilled to be building an incredible community of families around the world.

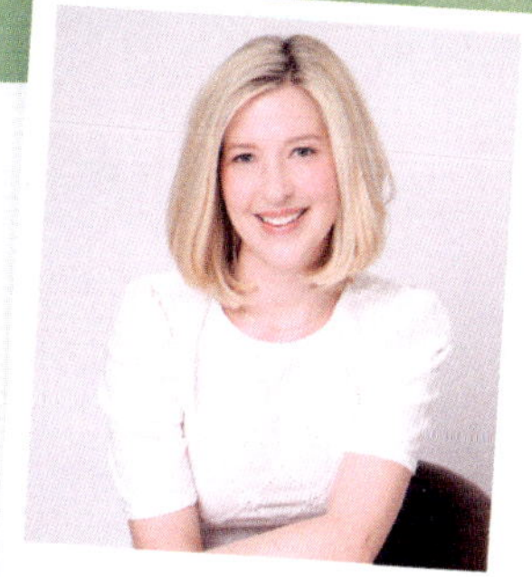

Cora Muccitelli

Illustrator

Cora is an illustrator and art director/designer based in Surrey, UK. With nearly two decades of design experience, this is her fourth illustrated book – a childhood aspiration since she first started drawing. Cora has two beautiful boys who bring her endless joy and is very grateful to have had Dr Golly's wisdom guiding her through motherhood. Working with the brand since inception, she has loved bringing his philosophy of empowering parents to life across all channels.

Your Baby Doesn't Come with a Book

The number-one bestselling, essential parenting guide for all first-time mums and dads.

There's no better parent for your baby than you!

Your Baby Doesn't Come with a Book covers EVERYTHING you need to know:

- Preparing your home
- What dads can do
- Understanding your baby's cues
- How to feed, settle, swaddle and bathe
- Plus – Dr Golly's famous active burping technique!

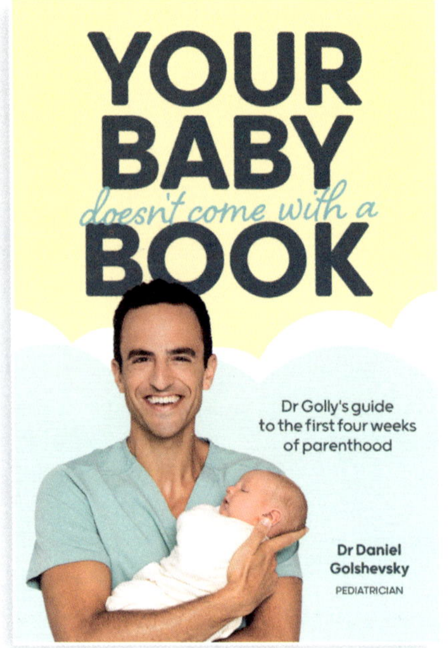

Dr Golly's books for children – out now!

Dr Golly's children's books are about two things core to his philosophy: reading your baby's cues and involving older children with the new baby.

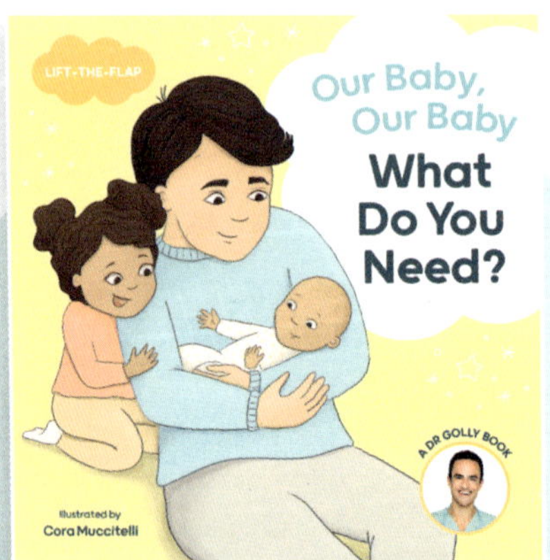

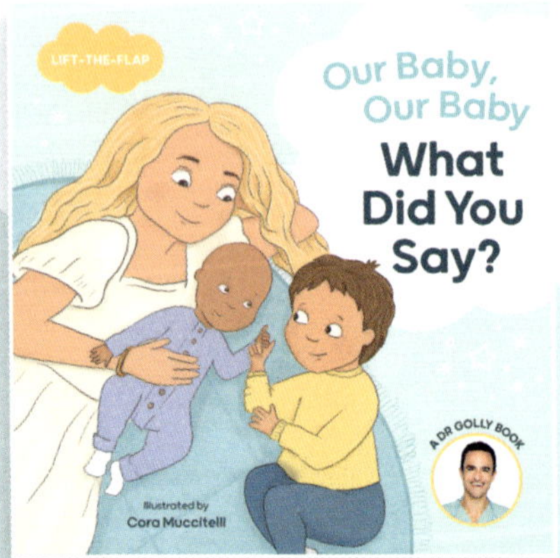

Shop Dr Golly's Sleep Programs

Continue your Dr Golly journey online:

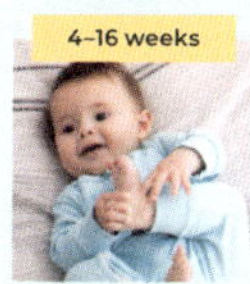

Little Baby Sleep Program

- Introducing a routine
- Aim to be sleeping from 11pm to 7am by 6 weeks

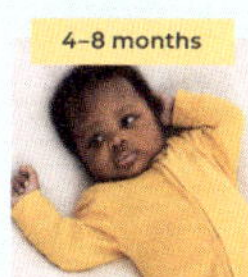

Big Baby Sleep Program

- Introducing solids and dropping night feeds
- Aim to be sleeping from 7pm to 7am by 6 months

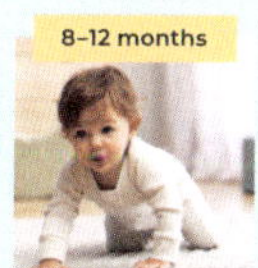

Pre-toddler Sleep Program

- Dropping to two daytime naps
- Starting daycare tips

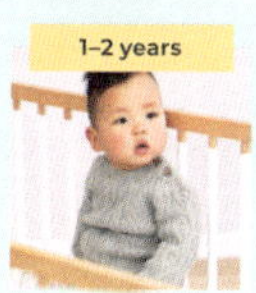

Toddler Sleep Program

- Dropping from two naps to one nap
- Settling techniques and parental alignment

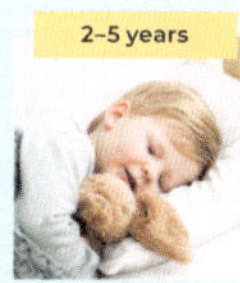

Pre-school Sleep Program

- Transitioning to a big bed
- Dropping day naps

drgolly.com

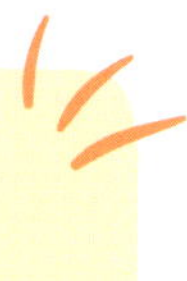

Scan here **to see if I have any discount offers or FREE bonuses for book readers!**

Dr Natasha Ching

Paediatric Infectious Diseases Physician

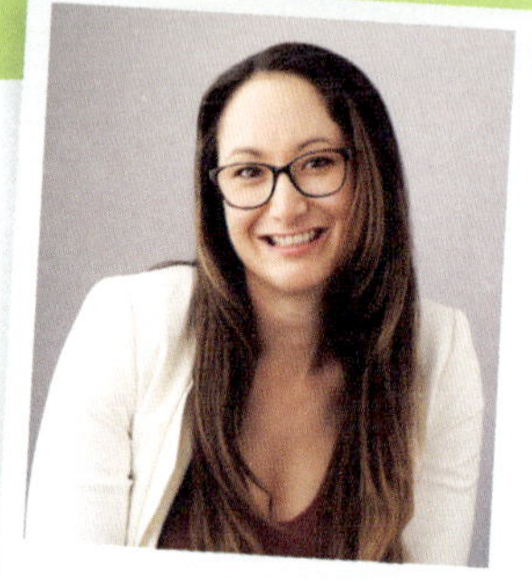

Natasha is a Paediatric Infectious Diseases Physician and General Paediatrician at Monash Children's Hospital, where she previously served as the Chief Resident Medical Officer. Throughout her career, she has been actively involved in research on childhood infections, contributing to numerous peer-reviewed publications. She has also reviewed and revised various hospital and state-wide guidelines and compiled a report for the World Health Organisation. As an Advanced Paediatric Life Support (APLS) instructor, she teaches healthcare professionals how to manage critically ill or injured children. Natasha is a proud mother of two with a goal to helping each child reach their fullest potential.

Background and Education:

- Bachelor of Medicine and Bachelor of Surgery, Monash University (Honours)
- Bachelor of Medical Sciences, Monash University (Honours)
- Fellow of The Royal Australasian College of Physicians

Dr Joseph Spencer

General Practitioner

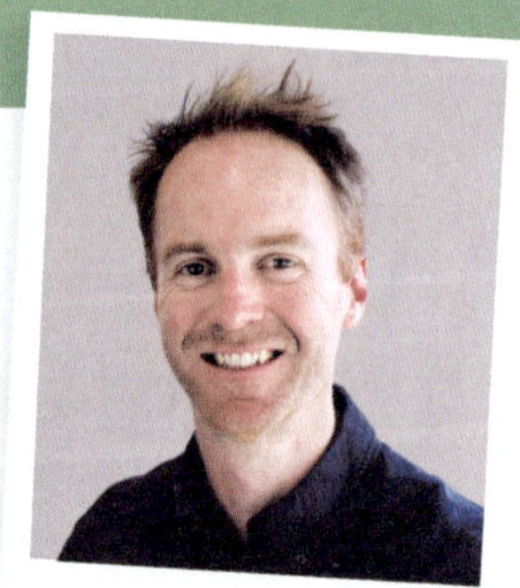

Dr Joe is a GP who works in a small coastal town and a father of two. He initially started his medical career as a Paramedic, but soon he realised he wanted to focus more on preventative health. He enjoys working with patients throughout their life cycle, from new families to acute injuries and chronic disease, and has a particular interest in skin cancer prevention and early treatment.

Background and Education:

- Bachelor of Emergency Health, Monash University (Dux)
- Ambulance Victoria Excellence Award, 2007
- Bachelor of Medicine & Surgery, Deakin University
- Fellow of the Royal Australian College of General Practitioners